Are You Ready to Get Your
Permanently Free From the Crip|

GW00374939

The**Migraine Cure**

How to Forever Banish the Curse of Migraines—
Using a Totally Effective, Safe, Clinically-Proven
Yet Drug-Free Medical Breakthrough.

SERGEY A. DZUGAN, MD, PHD

WITH DEBORAH MITCHELL

A LYNN SONBERG BOOK

The Migraine Cure

Published in the United States by:
Dragon Door Publications, Inc
P.O. Box 4381, St. Paul, MN 55104
Tel: (651) 487-2180
Fax: (651) 487-3954
Credit card orders: 1-800-899-5111
Email: support@dragondoor.com
Website: www.dragondoor.com

Book design, Illustrations and cover by Derek Brigham
Website http//www.dbrigham.com
Tel/Fax: (763) 208-3069 Email: dbrigham@visi.com

Manufactured in the United States
First Edition: November 2006

The Migraine Cure
Table of Contents

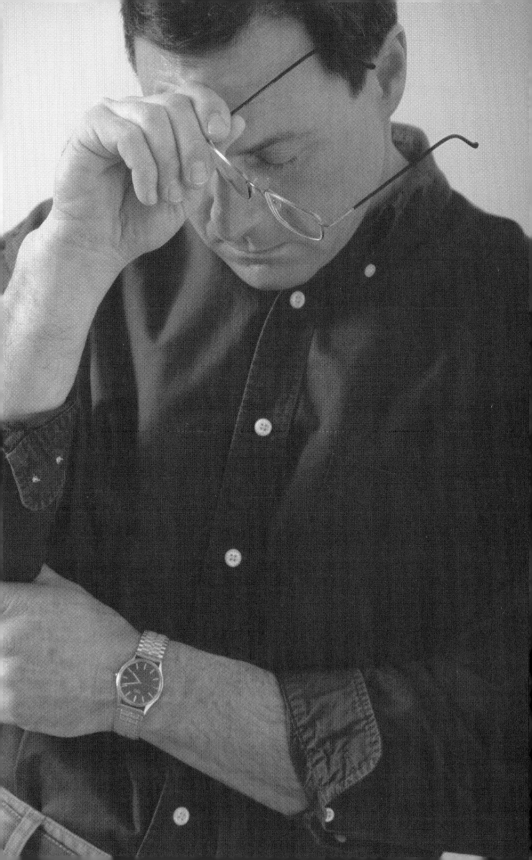

Introduction

I can only imagine what it's like to wake up each and every day and not know whether I will welcome the sun in my face or need to hide in a darkened room; not know whether I will relish the sound of children playing or need to seek a haven of silence; not know whether I will delight in sitting down to a fine meal with friends or need to sequester myself, nauseous and retching, away from those I love; not know whether I will be able to feel satisfaction after a day's work or need to cut short another day at the office.

Never did I imagine I would find a cure for migraine, a debilitating disease which, according to the National Headache Foundation, affects approximately 28 million Americans.

But I did.

I didn't set out to cure migraine. Like many groundbreaking medical events, the discovery happened serendipitously. In fact, I wasn't even working with migraine patients or in neurology at the time. Rather, before I came to the United States, I was Chief of Cardiovascular Surgery and the Senior Heart Surgeon at the Donetsk District Regional Hospital in the Ukraine. But it was here, while I was working with cancer patients at the North Central Mississippi Regional Cancer Center with R. Arnold Smith, MD, that something curious occurred. When cancer patients were treated with immunorestoration—a treatment approach that includes the use of hormones to help boost the immune system—patients who had once suffered with migraines reported that suddenly they were migraine-free. (We also noticed that high cholesterol was resolved, but that's another story.) Why were these patients suddenly free of migraine and its many related symptoms, including fatigue, insomnia, depression, and constipation? Could restoration of specific, foundational hormones be the basis of a migraine cure?

I had to know. Suddenly, I had an "incurable desire" to take on one of the most crippling conditions people can experience. Although as physicians we have a wide array of treatment options at our disposal—from moderate and heavy-hitting prescription pain killers to broadly tested herbal remedies—few doctors have been able to successfully treat, much less eliminate this condition for their patients. Until now, migraine has appeared to be impossible to cure. **But it's not impossible any more.**

Now There Is A Cure for Migraine

For the first time, there is a safe, proven cure for migraine headache and its associated symptoms. I developed the treatment protocol out of a long-term clinical study in which all the patients—100 percent—got complete relief from migraine pain and related symptoms, including individuals who had difficult-to-treat migraine that had plagued them for more than thirty years.

It seemed too good to be true, and you know what they say about such situations. But this was not a one-time occurrence. Since that study, I have repeatedly gotten the same results with hundreds of men, women, and adolescents in the United States and from around the world, whether they have been suffering with episodes of migraine pain for a few months or for decades. If they can find relief, you and your loved ones can find it as well. In the pages that follow, I share with you some of their success stories and how they achieved that success. More important, I explain how you can realize that success as well.

Some of the patients have called my treatment program a miracle. It is **not** a miracle: I do not wave a magic wand and make your migraine disappear. The treatment program is, however, soundly based in science, it is amazing, and it is effective. It is also natural, readily available, noninvasive, and fine-tuned for each individual to fit his or her unique needs.

Basically, I have developed a four-part program for migraine that is both simple and complex. I wanted it to be simple so people could understand it and follow it easily at home. This information is far too important to keep it out of the hands of everyone who needs it. The program's simplicity lies in the fact that the materials needed to achieve a cure are natural and readily accessible—hormones that are bioidentical to the body and which are available both over-the-counter and by prescription, as well as various nutrients or other natural supplements as needed, without prescription. You won't need to worry about taking drugs that will cause side effects or seeking the services of special practitioners or therapists; there aren't any medications in my program.

The program is also complex because each and every hormone, nutritional supplement, or other natural compound you may take as part of the plan has an intimate and critical relationship with all the others, and all the substances work together to achieve and maintain balance in what is called the sympathetic/ parasympathetic nervous systems. While it isn't necessary for you to have a thorough understanding of the equilibrium between the sympathetic and parasympathetic systems in order for you to benefit from the program, I do explain how this fascinating relationship works, with the aid of illustrations, because I believe it will provide you with a depth of appreciation not only of the migraine cure but of the intricate maneuverings required to achieve it.

A prominent professor has called my migraine treatment program "Nobel Prize material." Although it would be an honor to win such a prestigious prize, the real reward for me is the invaluable results it is providing the men, women, and young people who once suffered with migraine and who now are pain-free. I wrote this book so I could offer you the possibility of a cure. In the pages that follow, you will learn about how the program works, why it works, and, most important, how you can take the steps necessary to make it work for you—all without the use of expensive therapies or traditional drugs and the side effects associated with them.

How You Can Take Advantage of the Migraine Cure

Prior to publication of this book, the way most people heard about the Migraine Cure was through the nonprofit organization with which I am associated, Life Extension Foundation in Fort Lauderdale, Florida. The Foundation is, in a word, a **resource**, whose purpose is to provide the latest and relevant information on research from scientific and clinical studies to individuals and their health-care practitioners.

As president of Life Extension Scientific Information Inc., I supervise a staff of knowledgeable advisors who assist individuals who contact the Foundation in search information and ways to help them improve their health, extend human life, slow aging, prevent disease, and find the most effective therapies and remedies for their needs. No one on our staff forms a patient-physician relationship with any of the individuals who contact us, nor do they perform any type of physical examination, prescribe medications, or order tests or procedures. Once we provide people with information, they are encouraged to share it with their own health-care practitioners and to continue to seek additional information from the Foundation. We, in return, will continue to provide such assistance as long as people request it. If someone cannot find or does not have a health-care professional to consult, our advisors can provide a list of practitioners whom he or she can contact.

Among those who contact us are people with migraine who have read about the migraine management program in the articles I have written for the magazine published by the Foundation, and who heard about it by word of mouth. Good news, after all, does travel fast, and in this case it has circled the globe. When people with migraine contact the Foundation, I and my advisors explain how the Migraine Cure works, as I do in detail in this book. In fact, in this volume you will meet many of the individuals who have benefited from making that phone call. They learn that the migraine program is highly individualized and involves (1) undergoing a few blood tests, and (2) taking various natural supplements and bio-identical hormones (several of which must be obtained via prescription from your physician) on a daily basis.

And the rest, as they say, is history. Most people who carefully follow the recommendations of the Migraine Cure are migraine-free in as little as one week. One patient recently revealed to me that after she had been on the program for only two days, she conducted her own little "test" of the program: she ate something that had always triggered migraine in the past—a big dish of chocolate ice cream with chocolate sauce. Her results? Surprise—no migraine!

Here's wishing you many migraine-free years filled with all the goodness and sweetness life has to offer.

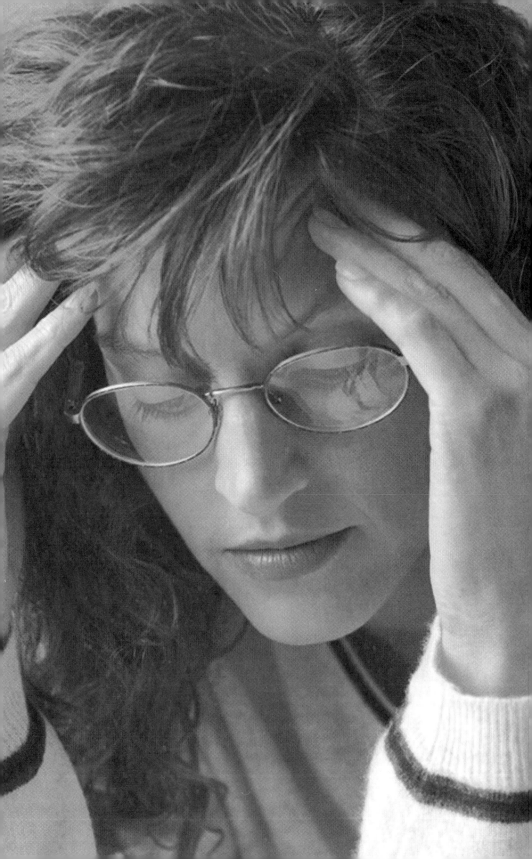

1

The Migraine Cure

Renee used to belong to an exclusive group, but belonging wasn't something she enjoyed or desired, even though such notables as Elvis Presley, John F. Kennedy, Vincent Van Gogh, and Sigmund Freud shared the distinction with her. That's because for nearly ten years, she counted herself among the more than 18 percent of the US population that experiences migraine. At least three or four days of each month she spent her days and nights in agony. She couldn't share time with her two children ages three and six, her husband, her friends, or her coworkers. The only time in the past ten years she had spent more than a few weeks without having a migraine was when she was pregnant. The migraines returned after each pregnancy and were still occurring regularly when she sought help from me after she heard about my program from a coworker.

"Skeptical, nervous, hopeful, curious, you name it, I felt it when I heard about this so-called migraine cure," said Renee. "But I was tired of taking medications, tired of the pain, the disruption to my life and the lives of my children and husband. I didn't want my kids to grow up hearing 'be quiet, mommy has a migraine' every few weeks."

Renee started the treatment program we developed for her the first week in February 2005. March came and went, then April and May. No migraine. By Thanksgiving Renee was giving thanks for ten migraine-free months. Now Renee is special for another reason: she is among the growing number of people who have rid themselves of migraine and its associated symptoms forever.

Migraine:
Millennia of Pain

"Not tonight, I have a headache" could very well have been uttered in the time of the ancient pharaohs, as archaeologists have unearthed headache prescriptions written on papyrus. Hippocrates (470-410 BC), the father of medicine, believed that sexual intercourse or exercise could trigger a headache and that vomiting could provide some relief. Indeed, many migraine and headache patients do feel better once they vomit. Although people in the time of the pharaohs and Hippocrates likely experienced migraines, it wasn't until around 150 AD that someone assigned a specific name for this special type of head pain that typically occurs on one side of the head. The term "migraine" is derived from the Greek word "hemicrania" (half-skull), which describes the one-sided nature of migraine, and was introduced by Galen, a well-known Roman experimental physiologist. Galen believed migraine was caused by excessive vapors, either too cold or too hot, that rose from the stomach to the head. Given that our ancient ancestors did not have the technology we have today, nor the benefit of centuries of knowledge, we cannot fault Galen on his guess.

Fast forward nearly two millennia, and, until now, the medical community still does not fully understand what causes migraine, nor how to treat it effectively. In fact, the modern approach to treating migraine is typically attributed to Pat Humphrey and his associates, who developed the drug sumatriptan, a chemical that is similar to serotonin, a neurotransmitter that is produced naturally in the body and found in large concentrations in the brain. (We will learn more about the role of serotonin in migraine later in this chapter.) Once Humphrey's team discovered that serotonin could relieve headache, the race was on to develop drugs that performed similarly to serotonin and sumatriptan.

Today numerous pharmaceutical companies have developed drugs that fall into the drug classification called triptans, which contains medications similar to sumatriptan. These drugs are somewhat effective in relieving migraine and some of its related symptoms in some patients some of the time, and they are far from a cure. Not exactly a ringing endorsement.

Migraine:
What is it?

Researchers and medical experts have told the public many things about migraine and migraineurs (the term for people who suffer with migraine) over the years. Migraineurs themselves have much to tell us as well, and in fact I have found that listening to their individual stories is absolutely critical when they seek treatment, because each and every person reveals unique characteristics and experiences that can help when it comes to developing the best way to apply the treatment program—the Migraine Cure — to his or her needs. Although laboratory test results are an essential part of the treatment approach, they must be weighed along with personal, emotional, and social factors. The Migraine Cure is not about eliminating symptoms or curing disease; it's about restoring balance, health, and quality of life, and in the process, migraine disappears.

CHARACTERISTICS OF MIGRAINE

That being said, there are some basic facts about migraines that hold true for the condition in general. These include the following:

- Migraine is a disease that has many symptoms, the primary one being a pulsing or throbbing pain that typically, but not exclusively, occurs on one side of the head.

- Migraine is accompanied by nausea in about 80 percent of episodes, vomiting in about 30 percent, extreme sensitivity to light (photophobia) in about 90 percent, and extreme sensitivity to sound (phonophobia) in about 80 percent.

- Migraineurs often experience and/or have been diagnosed with other health conditions, including fibromyalgia, fatigue (including chronic fatigue syndrome), confusion, sinusitis, asthma, eczema, irritable bowel, itchy bumps on the skin, muscle and joint pain, urinary tract symptoms, agitation, sleep disorders, stiff or tender neck, lightheadedness, and tender scalp.

- Up to half the people who have migraines experience a "warning" that an attack is imminent. This is also known as a "prodrome" and is not the same as an aura (see below). This warning can develop gradually over a 24-hour period and include symptoms such as irritability, yawning a lot, difficulty speaking, and craving certain foods.

- Frequency of migraine can range from a once in a lifetime to almost daily. Overall, 38 percent of migraineurs have from one to 12 attacks per year; 37 percent have one to three per month, 11 percent experience one per week, and 14 percent suffer with two to six migraines per week.

- A minority of migraineurs experience an aura—a sensory or visual disturbance, such as flashing lights or zig-zag images, or tingling and/or numbness in an arm or on the side of the face— about 15 to 30 minutes before onset of the head pain. Some individuals also feel confused or weak. This type of migraine is called "migraine with aura" (formerly called "classic migraine").

- Most migraineurs (about 80%) do not experience an aura; this type of migraine is called "migraine without aura" (formerly called "common migraine").

- Generally, the headache phase lasts from 2 hours to 2 days in children and 4 hours to three days in adults if left untreated or if treated unsuccessfully.

- Migraineurs are many times more likely than headache-free individuals to develop major depression.

- Migraine episodes can be triggered by various stimuli, both internal and external, and any one individual may respond to different triggers at different times. In fact, 85 percent of migraineurs report triggers, and most are affected by more than one, with three being the mean number. I discuss triggers in more detail below, but here I want to emphasize that these triggers *do not cause* migraine.

- Rather, "triggers" are exactly what their name implies: they set into motion an underlying physiological propensity for something in the body to malfunction. In the case of migraine, triggers have an impact on an existing biochemical imbalance in the body that then initiates the physiological chain reaction that results in migraine.

- Migraine affects approximately 28 million Americans, and 75 percent of those who get migraine are women. The one-year prevalence of migraine is 18 percent in women, 6 percent in men, and 5 percent among children. The lifetime prevalence is 25 percent for women and 8 percent for men.

- Most people who suffer with migraine do not seek medical care and/or have not been diagnosed by a physician and instead treat themselves with over-the-counter and/or alternative remedies (see chapter 3). Reasons for this failure to seek medical care include high cost of prescription medications and the ineffectiveness and/or side effects associated with prescription drugs.

- Chronic or frequent migraines can increase the risk of stroke. One recent study (2005), for example, shows that the risk of stroke doubles for migraine sufferers, while another notes that women with migraine with aura have a greater than 50 percent increased risk of total stroke and 70 percent increased risk of ischemic stroke compared with women who do not have migraine.

- Migraine is a huge burden on the economy: it cost taxpayers $13 billion in missed work and decreased productivity per year in the United States.

- Until now, no one has definitively identified the causes of migraine and correlated an appropriate course of treatment to eliminate it.

Triggers

For people who suffer with migraine, a trigger is a substance, activity, environmental stimulus, or other factor that either initiates or contributes to an existing hormonal and/or metabolic imbalance that eventually manifests as migraine symptoms. Migraine triggers can be things you can control or things you cannot, and many people respond to both types.

One of the symptoms of migraine is hypersensitivity of the senses. Many migraineurs are so exquisitely sensitive to light and/or sound that they must retreat to a darkened, quiet place when they are having an attack. In addition to light and sound, both of which are largely controllable triggers, others in this category include strong or unusual odors, touch, changes in

---

Foods Identified As Possible Triggers of Migraine

- Alcoholic beverages, especially redwine
- Aspartame (name brands include Equal, NutraSweet)
- Avocados
- Beans (including broad, lima, garbanzo, Italian, navy, pinto)
- Brewer's yeast
- Caffeine
- Cheese (aged)
- Chocolate
- Dairy products (cultured, such as buttermilk, sour cream)
- Figs
- Lentils
- Meats (aged, cured, or processed, such as bologna, hot dogs, herring, pepperoni)
- Monosodium glutamate (MSG) including meat tenderizer
- Nuts
- Onions
- Papaya
- Passion fruit
- Peanut butter
- Pea pods
- Pickled or marinated foods (pickles, olives, snack foods, sauerkraut)
- Raisins
- Red plums
- Seasoned salt
- Snow peas
- Soups (canned or bouillon cubes)
- Soy sauce

sleeping habits or amount of sleep, intense physical activity (including sexual activity), stress, secondhand smoke, use of birth control pills, missing meals, and certain foods, especially those that contain tyramine, sodium nitrate, or phenylalanine.

Among uncontrollable triggers, the most important and common one is menstruation, which involves significant hormonal fluctuations. (The first trimester of pregnancy is another uncontrollable trigger situation, as this is when estrogen levels change drastically.) Sixty to 70 percent of women report migraine or a severe headache within seven to ten days of beginning menstruation. And because it involves fluctuations in hormones—and the Migraine Cure is about balancing hormones—this "uncontrollable" trigger can be defused when we make appropriate adjustments to a woman's hormone levels and the ratios between them. I talk a great deal more about hormone balancing in chapter 4.

Uncontrollable triggers include changes in the weather (temperature, wind, barometric pressure, humidity) and altitude. Some people, for example, experience more migraine attacks in the summer while others are more affected by high humidity and rainy weather.

Regardless of the number or type of triggers that affect you, it is possible to completely disarm them with the Migraine Cure. Bettina, who lived with relentless migraines nearly every other day for 48 years, tells how her former triggers just disappeared once she restored hormonal and metabolic balance with the Migraine Cure. "I have gone through root canals, garage sales, changes in barometric pressure, changes in altitude, eating chocolate, bright flashy lights, drinking a gin and tonic and a glass or two or wine— all things that would have triggered a migraine in the past — with no migraines," she said. "I am amazed that this is working for me."

Some studies have shown that some migraineurs get relief, usually temporary, if they eliminate known triggers of migraine. However, if they do not balance their hormones and nervous system functions, the propensity or underlying cause of migraine will still be there even if they eliminate the migraine triggers. The fact is, once we balance the hormones and the sympathetic and parasympathetic nervous systems, substances and situations that were once triggers for migraine are not triggers any longer.

Not Migraine: Cluster Headache

Although the focus of this book is migraine, I am including cluster headache as part of our discussion because it also responds to hormone restoration and the other elements of the Migraine Cure. In chapter 5, for example, you'll read about how cluster headaches respond well to the pineal gland restoration part of the treatment program.

Of perhaps more than passing interest is that while migraines are much more common in women, cluster headaches occur primarily in men by a margin of 6 to 1. This debilitating head pain typically affects one side of the head and is characterized by a stabbing pain behind one eye, which usually waters profusely. Nasal congestion, nausea, and sweating are also common symptoms. Stabbing pain may awaken the individual at night or begin at the same time each day. According to the American Academy of Family Physicians, cluster headaches usually last for 30 to 45 minutes, but can last a few minutes or several hours. They typically occur at the same time each day, and this pattern may last for four to eight weeks and recur every few months or go into remission for years.

Although conventional medicine practitioners place cluster headache into the "cause unknown" category, there are several theories about its causes, and as with migraine, several of them point to hormone imbalance as well as disruption between the sympathetic and parasympathetic nervous systems. For example, some experts note that cluster headache is characterized by effects of the sympathetic (forehead sweating) and parasympathetic (eye tearing, nasal congestion, runny nose) nervous systems. It is also a fact that cluster headache often recur at the same time every day, which suggests that the hypothalamus, which controls hormone secretion and circadian rhythms, may play a major role. Fluctuations in serotonin levels are also seen in cluster headache.

Migraine:
The Misunderstood Malady

We've been told that migraine is a primary disorder, meaning it is a condition that is not caused by other underlying medical conditions. Indeed, researchers have approached their search for migraine's cause with this idea in mind. Treating migraine would be so much easier if it were true: One cause, one recommended course of treatment. What we have instead, however, is a long list of theories about what causes this malady (see details below, "What 'They' Say Causes Migraine"). These theories are important, as they provide a treasure trove of information, and there is scientific data that support each one of them. However, the fact is, no single theory adequately explains the underlying cause of migraine nor explains all the laboratory findings and observations researchers and other professionals have made over the years about migraine.

What "They" Say Causes Migraine

More than a dozen theories have been put forth as to what causes migraine. Rather than discuss all of them, let's look at the ones that made the most significant contributions to the development of the Migraine Cure program.

- **Blood vessel constriction and dilation.** This is probably the most well-known theory associated with migraine, and it is one of the first ever proposed as well. In the early 1850s, two French scientists, Brown-Sequard and Claude Bernard, proposed that dilated blood vessels (vasodilation) in the brain were the cause of migraine pain. Less than a decade later, however, a German physiologist, Emil Du Bois-Reymond, proposed that constriction of the brain's blood vessels (vasoconstriction) was the cause. Both theories involve an abnormal flow of blood in the brain, which indeed is common among migraineurs but does not occur in all migraine patients. However, blood vessel constriction and dilation are believed to be factors in migraine. In fact, some physicians prescribe vasoconstricting drugs called ergots (see details in chapter 4) for some of their migraine patients.

- **Steroid hormone influence.** There is significant evidence that steroid hormones (e.g., the estrogens, progesterone, testosterone, DHEA, pregnenolone, cortisol) play a major role in migraine. Support for this theory can be seen in, for example, the fact that migraine affects approximately three times as many women as men; migraine attacks occur during menstruation in 60 percent of women; and use of oral contraceptives affect the incidence and severity of migraine. The impact of these hormones on the body and migraine in particular is complex as well as exciting, and I explore it in detail in chapters 2 and 4. Here I want to note, however, that although many investigators have conducted studies in which they administered these hormones to manage migraine, their results have not been consistent. My work with steroid hormones, which lead to the Migraine Cure, uncovered the main problem with these studies and thus has been 100 percent consistent and 100 percent effective in eliminating migraine.

- **Serotonin effect.** We know that the body's level of a brain chemical called serotonin declines during a migraine attack. It's also known that the level of serotonin in the urine increases during a migraine, which indicates that the body is releasing a large amount of the chemical. Serotonin regulates pain signals in the brain and along many pain pathways, including the trigeminal nerve system. Some experts believe that when serotonin levels drop during headache, this triggers the trigeminal nerve (the largest of the cranial nerves, it runs throughout the face and head) to release chemicals called neuropeptides, which travel to the brain's outer covering and cause the blood vessels to become inflamed, resulting in migraine pain. Thus many physicians prescribe drugs that selectively stimulate certain serotonin receptors. These drugs, collectively called triptans (see chapter 3) reduce the symptoms of migraine. Serotonin also plays another role in migraine, as you'll see below under "Impaired pineal gland function."

- **Genetic predisposition.** According to the American Council for Headache Education and various experts, up to 90 percent of migraineurs have a family history of the disorder. In addition, recent studies have identified several genes that appear to predispose some individuals to migraine. The presence of these genes seems to cause dysfunction in ion transport of sodium and potassium and to influence calcium transport between cells, all of which are involved in migraine, as you will learn later in chapter 7. More recent (January 2006) research has focused on the possible presence of genes that influence the blood vessels (vascular) and hormone levels and functioning as having a role in migraine susceptibility. This possibility is under investigation.

- **Hyperexcitable brain.** An imbalance in brain biochemistry can result in a hyperexcitable brain, in which there is abnormal neuron (nerve cell) activity. Such activity can be caused by several different conditions, including low levels of magnesium in the brain, mitochondrial abnormalities, dysfunctions related to increased levels of nitric oxide (increased nitric oxide production causes arteries to dilate and thus migraine can occur), or a type of calcium channelopathy, a disease that involves dysfunction of the calcium ions such as familial hemiplegic migraine. If this all seems confusing now, it will become clearer later when I discuss the Migraine Cure in detail in chapters 4 through 7. Drugs that address the hyperexcitable brain theory include anticonvulsants, which are prescribed to help prevent migraine (see chapter 3).

- **Impaired pineal gland function.** This gland, located deep in the brain, harbors the neurotransmitter serotonin and melatonin, another hormone that plays a role in migraine and that we'll be discussing in detail later. The relationship between serotonin and melatonin is critical, as serotonin is the precursor of melatonin; that is, it is the substance from which melatonin is produced. Therefore, low serotonin levels result in low melatonin levels as well, and we know melatonin is low in migraineurs.

So What IS Migraine?

So what is migraine if it is not a primary disorder caused by any one of the factors listed? I propose that migraine is not a single disorder, but a collection of disorders; specifically, the consequence or result of an intricate combination of neurohormonal and metabolic imbalances. What this means—as my research and experience have shown me again and again—is that in some individuals, an imbalance in the levels of certain hormones (namely, the estrogens, progesterone, testosterone, DHEA, and pregnenolone), along with dysfunction of the pineal gland and its hormone production and an imbalance in metabolic functioning work together to cause the head pain and symptoms associated with the disease of migraine.

The bottom line: migraine is a very complex condition, but once you understand the imbalances that contribute to it, the remedy becomes apparent.

"Sizing Up" an Effective Migraine Treatment Plan

Once I discovered that an imbalance of hormones and metabolism was the combination of factors behind migraine, I set out to fine-tune a treatment plan. Without going into an indepth explanation of the plan—which I do in the following chapters—here I want to note an important feature of the Migraine Cure: one size does not fit all. Unlike the current drug treatment approach to migraine, my recommendations do not involve prescribing "Drug A" to everyone who feels a migraine coming on, and "Drug B" to everyone who experiences symptoms. The Migraine Cure is based on a basic concept — balancing the function of specific systems in the body— and tailoring the dosing of specific hormones and other natural substances to meet the unique needs of each individual.

If you want to eliminate your migraine, you and a competent health-care professional need to identify your current level of various hormones and nutrients, including your calcium-to-magnesium ratio; establish the functioning status of your pineal gland and digestive/intestinal tract; and then choose which natural, biocompatible supplements you will need to restore all of your levels and functions to their natural, healthy state. All this is done without the use of drugs or expensive therapies.

The Conventional Approach: Treat Symptoms

When Jonathan talked to me about his migraine, he shared an all-too-familiar tale. He had been suffering with migraines for more than a decade and had spent at least eight of those years living on prescription medications. He told me how he averaged one to two migraines per week and had sought help from seven different doctors. Every doctor told him the same thing: keep taking medication. So he did. Jonathan estimated that he had given himself hundreds of sumatriptan injections and taken thousands of doses of other drugs, both prescription and over-the-counter. Sometimes he got significant relief; other times he did not. Sometimes he got sufficient warning so he could ward off the worst of the pain with medication; other times the pain hit before he could take precautions. Jonathan was convinced he would be facing these challenges for the rest of his life.

Fortunately, Jonathan learned about the Migraine Cure and within one month of starting the program, he was completely migraine-free. (You'll meet Jonathan again and learn more about his treatment program later in the book.) But that's only because the Migraine Cure addresses the causes of migraine and tailors treatment for each individual. This differs from the prevention and treatment approach currently taken by the conventional medical establishment, which addresses symptoms only and addresses them primarily through use of medications. Doctors treat migraine based on what they believe the underlying cause to be. As we saw above under "What They Say Causes Migraine," each theory of the cause of migraine comes with its own treatment plan. The problem is, no single treatment approach works for every person, and the same approach doesn't even always work for each migraine episode an individual has.

Although medication is the main way migraine is treated in the United States, it is by no means the only approach. We will take a closer look at various current prevention and treatment therapies for migraine—both conventional and alternative/complementary — and why they don't work in chapter 3.

Why We Can Cure Migraine—Now

Quite simply, we can cure migraine now because we know the underlying mechanisms of this serious disorder and how to correct them. The Migraine Cure addresses each of these factors and incorporates a strategy to restore balance among all the systems involved in migraine. Migraine is a complex condition that requires a multidimensional approach; it cannot be cured with a single medication, herb, nutritional supplement, or integrative therapy technique. The good news about this approach is that all the elements are natural, bio-friendly, readily available, virtually without side effects, and most important, effective.

Let me share with you one of the studies I and my colleague did that lead us to the Migraine Cure. At this point I will not go into a detailed explanation of each of the steps; that I save until later chapter. For now it's just important that you get an idea of just how powerful this treatment approach is.

In this study, which ran from May 2001 to May 2004, we offered our migraine program to 21 women and 2 men who ranged in age from 29 to 66 years. All of them had tried unsuccessfully to prevent and/or treat migraine for a period ranging from 2 to 36 years and had used as many as four conventional drugs in the process. Nearly three-quarters (73.9%) of the patients had used hormone replacement therapy or oral contraceptives at some point, but without adequate relief. Along with migraine, all of the patients complained of fatigue, 95.7 percent reported depression, 82.6 percent had insomnia, and 21.7 percent had fibromyalgia. These are conditions that commonly appear in people who suffer with migraine.

We held detailed consultations with each patient, gathered information on medical and personal history, and then administered routine blood tests to determine a baseline lipid (cholesterol) profile as well as levels of steroid hormones: pregnenolone, DHEA sulfate, progesterone, total estrogen (females) or estradiol (males), and total testosterone. Overall, the results showed that every patient had deficiencies of the steroid hormones, with a deficiency of pregnenolone being the most prominent. Based on the information gathered and the test results, we then developed a comprehensive treatment program for each patient, based on his or her individual needs, that included:

- Hormone restoration therapy using bio-identical hormones in specially prepared formulations that ensure the body utilizes them properly (details on dosing appears in chapter 4): oral pregnenolone and DHEA, transdermal estrogens (90% estriol, 7% estradiol, and 3% estrone), micronized progesterone gel, and testosterone gel.

- Rebalancing the function of the pineal gland using melatonin, kava root extract, and vitamin B6 at bedtime. I discuss this further in chapter 5.

- Rebalancing of the magnesium to calcium ratio by giving magnesium citrate at bedtime.

- Improving the function of the digestive system, including better absorption of nutrients and restoration of a healthy level of intestinal flora with the use of probiotics (microorganisms that help maintain the health of the intestinal tract), including organisms in the *Lactobacillus and Bifidobacterium* groups.

I discuss the treatment program in greater detail in later chapters, but for now let me cut to the chase: we had a 100 percent success rate. No patient suffered a migraine after he or she started the program, even those who had lived with migraine for decades. In addition, symptoms of fatigue, depression, insomnia, and fibromyalgia also disappeared, and no patient had any significant side effects or complications associated with treatment.

How fast can you expect relief if you try the Migraine Cure? Patients who follow the treatment plan as it is recommended for their specific needs can be migraine free within one week of starting treatment. The secret? There is no secret, just a willingness to follow the treatment plan. The plan, as you'll see in the stories that I share with you throughout the rest of this book, involves taking various supplements throughout the day according to your body's biorhythms. It may seem a bit bothersome at first, but remember: your body is out of balance, and we attempt to restore balance, which means we must follow nature's course.

In Conclusion

Quite simply, there is a cure for migraine. For Bettina, who did not take part in the study but who learned about the migraine program later, the cure didn't come a moment too soon. (You'll read about Bettina later in the book.) After suffering with migraines for nearly fifty years, she was "amazed that this [Migraine Cure] is working for me. I thought I was beyond hope. Conventional medicine and conventional doctors are just not on the same page yet. We [migraineurs] don't have time to wait for them. Our lives are going by now."

And with that introduction, let's begin to explore the Migraine Cure.

2

Four Steps To A Cure

If I had to use one word to describe my approach to the successful treatment and elimination of migraine, that word would be **balance.** The approach involves an orchestrated and synchronized adjustment of the components and functions of several systems in the body (described below) to achieve that goal. But this is no standard balancing act. To be successful, we need to evaluate the unique needs of each individual who has migraine, plus measure and assess the components and functions of the various systems involved using the data gathered from a thorough history, results of blood tests, and information from ongoing evaluations. Based on our findings, we can then recommend the most appropriate natural hormones and supplements to restore balance, make dosage adjustments as needed along the way, and thus eliminate migraine.

Based on our research and clinical experience, including the study I discussed in chapter 1, we called our approach the Neurohormonal and Metabolic Dysbalance Hypothesis of Migraine (aka, the Migraine Cure), which for the first time identifies the crucial relationship among the components that together play the defining roles in the development, occurrence, and treatment of migraine. The various components and biochemical functions that are involved in migraine and the Migraine Cure have a complex and fascinating relationship that includes dozens, if not hundreds of balancing acts between hormones, enzymes, nutrients, the functions of glands and organs, and other factors. I have tried to simplify this relationship by breaking it down into four general "steps" or areas that we address in the

Migraine Cure. (These are not "steps" in the traditional sense, because we do not first address one, then another, and so on, but more like components, which are initiated and addressed simultaneously.) Keep in mind that there is constant communication between the components in each of these areas and so sometimes the "lines" between them are not distinct. Those areas are as follows:

- **Neurohormonal system:** This area includes the activities of the hypothalamus, the pituitary gland, and the glands that produce steroid hormones, namely the ovaries, testes, and adrenal glands. Our goal is to restore the hormones that are produced by these glands to levels that **are appropriate for the individual.** These levels are different for each person, and so the recommended doses of various hormones for each patient can vary significantly from one person to another.

- **Pineal gland:** This gland balances the cyclic production of the neurotransmitter serotonin and the hormone melatonin, both of which are key players in migraine, so our goal here is to reset the function of the pineal gland. As I mentioned previously, serotonin is the precursor of melatonin, thus the relationship between these substances is an important one to watch. To help achieve and maintain an optimal balance between the pineal gland's function and the rest of the Migraine Cure, we frequently add the herb kava root to a patient's program.

- **Digestive system:** Harmony in the digestive tract includes achieving a healthy intestinal flora that promotes regular elimination and proper absorption of nutrients, which we have found is essential for avoidance of migraine. Given that 70 percent of migraineurs also have some type of gastrointestinal disorder, restoration of balance within the digestive system is a critical part of the Migraine Cure. We have found, for example, that constipation, which most migraineurs experience, **must** be resolved in order to eliminate migraine.

- **Magnesium balance:** Another factor in this part of the program is achieving a balance between two critical minerals—magnesium and calcium—as an imbalance between these substances can change the electrical activity of the cell membranes which, as you'll soon learn, is a crucial factor in migraine.

- **Sympathetic and parasympathetic systems:** As we work to balance the four systems mentioned above, we are also simultaneously working toward a balance between the sympathetic and parasympathetic nervous systems, which is the ultimate goal of the Migraine Cure. I explain the basics of the sympathetic and parasympathetic nervous systems later in this chapter, but here I just want to mention that a balance between these two systems is critical for prevention of migraine and, indeed, several other medical maladies, which you'll learn more about in chapter 7.

The critical point I need to mention here is that **all these components are intimately related and work together, and so it is absolutely essential that the first four systems be addressed together so we achieve a balance between the sympathetic and parasympathetic systems.** For example, when we recommend specific doses of estrogen and progesterone to restore hormonal balance between these hormones, it also helps restore balance between the sympathetic and parasympathetic nervous systems. Similarly, when we suggest specific calcium and magnesium supplements to restore the proper balance between these two minerals, we also are bringing harmony to the sympathetic and parasympathetic nervous systems.

Participating in the Migraine Cure is like taking care of your car. Your car needs thousands of parts and dozens of fluids and other substances to keep it running properly. If you decide to replace only a few of the needed parts or fluids when they are damaged or deficient, the car won't run properly. Would you put air into just two tires and not the other two and expect the car to run well? Similarly, in the Migraine Cure we need to balance all the steroid hormone levels and address specific other hormone, nutrient, metabolic, and system needs, not just one or two. All of the systems and changes that occur within them are interrelated, and any one or more of the changes can trigger migraine. Patients who have carefully followed the recommendations of the Migraine Cure have become migraine-free, some for the first time in decades.

Many of the words and concepts I've just mentioned here, like "neurohormonal," "pineal gland," "neurotransmitter," "sympathetic," and "parasympathetic" may mean little or nothing to you, but I assure you that by the time you reach the end of this chapter, you will come to appreciate the incredible roles they play in creating balance in your body. You will also come to realize how maintaining a harmonious relationship between the sympathetic and parasympathetic nervous systems is the key factor in whether you will get rid of your migraine forever.

Overview Of The Migraine Cure

In this section I explain how the different components of the Migraine Cure work together to eliminate migraine. This is what might be called the "nuts and bolts" of the program, as it looks at the relationship among the various components at a cellular level. You might ask, "Is it necessary for me to understand all the biochemistry behind the Migraine Cure in order to benefit from it?" or more to the point, "Dr. Dzugan, can I skip this chapter and get right to the program?"

No, you don't **need** to understand the biochemistry of the program, but many patients have told me that they enjoy learning about what makes the Migraine Cure "tick." "I discovered how truly complicated and yet fascinating the whole migraine phenomenon is once I learned how it develops and then what it takes to eliminate it," said one patient. "I couldn't believe there were so many interrelated components to migraine," said another former migraineur. "Each component is like a family member, trying to get along with another member. And the goal of the program is harmony, not a feud, just like in a real family."

Yes, you can skip this chapter and proceed to chapters 4 through 7. But I and many former migraineurs urge you to read through this information, as it will help you better appreciate much of what is involved in the development and elimination of migraine. Also, although the basic treatment program is not complicated, it typically requires adjustments in dosing and in adding or stopping certain hormones or supplements along the way. I find, and patients are quick to agree with me, that having a fuller understanding of the underlying reasons and functions of the different steps and supplements allows patients to feel more in control of their treatment and encourages them to ask questions and interact more easily with whomever they work with, which in turn can make their recovery much smoother and faster.

THE MIGRAINE CURE IN A NUTSHELL

No two people with migraine are alike; each person comes looking for help with has his or her own symptom profile, concomitant medical conditions, medication and other treatment history, family history, expectations, and diet, exercise, and other lifestyle habits. But while I approach each migraineur as an individual who has unique needs, I also apply a specific set of guidelines and treatment strategies that I developed, tested, and retested. Thus, in a nutshell, here is what happens when someone wants to begin the Migraine Cure (Individuals are advised to talk to their physician before starting any type of treatment. Several of the hormones in the Migraine Cure require a doctor's prescription).

- An individual hears or reads about the migraine program and contacts Life Extension Foundation, where he or she can talk to or correspond with one of the advisors on my team and learn about how the program works (If you are interested in learning more about the Migraine Cure program as described in this book, you can contact Dr. Sergey Dzugan and his medical staff at 1-877-402-2721 or at www.fountain-migraine.com).

- An advisor conducts an in-depth interview to gather information about the individual's personal and family history and current health status.

- An advisor suggests the individual undergo blood tests to identify lipid and hormone levels. The tests are done at the convenience of the patient, and the results are sent to Life Extension Foundation for evaluation.

- An advisor reviews the test results with the individual and suggests a detailed program. At this time the advisor will recommend that the migraineur stop taking any supplements (but NOT medications) he or she is using for the duration of the migraine program, which typically lasts for two to three months.

- The migraineur begins hormone restoration therapy, digestive therapy, magnesium supplementation, and pineal gland recharging.

- The individual withdraws from all migraine-related medications within a few days of starting the program if he or she has not done so already.

- The migraineur is encouraged to maintain close communication with his or her advisor so the program can be monitored and modifications can be made as needed

- If the individual follows the plan as outlined, he or she can expect to be migraine-free within as little as a few days. Relief from migraine-related symptoms, such as fatigue, insomnia, gastrointestinal problems, mood swings, aches and pains, and depression also often become evident within a few days of beginning the program.

- If individuals follow the program as recommended, they typically can stop or dramatically reduce the number and/or dose of any supplements they have been taking as part of the program.

Getting To Know You

When you go to a doctor's office for the first time, you can expect to fill out a patient history form where you list family health history, your past and current health condition, medical procedures and surgeries, allergies, and medication use. This is all important data, but the information needed to effectively implement the Migraine Cure typically goes deeper—and is more personal — than that. Sometimes the small clues that are revealed during the interviewing process are the most helpful.

Melissa is a good example. She had spent the last eight of her forty-six years fighting monthly migraines that kept her bedridden and suffering with nausea and vomiting for at least two to three days each episode. Melissa had been a high-level manager at an advertising firm, but eventually the stress of her job and the severity of the migraines made it impossible for her to function effectively, and she quit, although she did some consulting work occasionally.

Melissa revealed that in addition to migraine, she also had a history of chronic fatigue syndrome, severe depression, sleep problems, osteoporosis, anorexia (during her teen years), severe mood swings, and premenstrual syndrome. Her menstrual cycle was regular at 28 days. She said she had no sex drive and had in fact not been sexually active for several years because of loss of libido and vaginal dryness.

The first step was for Melissa to undergo a complete female hormone panel (which reveals the levels of all three estrogens, progesterone, total testosterone, pregnenolone, and dehydroepiandrosterone sulfate [DHEA-S]) and a lipid profile. When her results came back, all the levels were within the normal range except for slightly elevated total cholesterol and slightly low DHEA-S. Her pregnenolone level, which is virtually always abnormal in migraineurs, was normal. Clearly we needed to look further, and that's when something Melissa said during her interview took on new importance: she said that before the migraines began at age 37, she had had excess body hair, including some upper lip hair, very hairy legs, and hairs on her breasts. Immediately before the migraines began, however, the excess body hair decreased significantly.

The excess body hair was a sign that she had testosterone dominance. It appeared that for Melissa, a testosterone level that was slightly higher than normal **for the general population** was normal for her. Therefore, we needed to restore her hormones to levels that were uniquely suited for her. Once we did, her migraines disappeared, her sex drive reappeared, and her depression lifted.

Melissa is just one example of how important it is to gather information that conventional history taking procedures do not include or do not find relevant. The presence of facial hair in women, for example, indicates a dominance of testosterone, while women who are experiencing fibroids, endometriosis, irregular menstrual cycles, or moodiness may very likely find they have a deficiency of progesterone. Another example is constipation. This symptom is very common among migraineurs and is one that **must** be resolved if migraine is to be eliminated. Constipation is also an indication that an individual has a dominance of the sympathetic nervous system activity at night, which means we need to identify the imbalance and then recommend the appropriate agents to restore harmony. We discuss digestive and intestinal balance in chapter 6.

Once an individual agrees to follow the program, he or she must agree to stop all prescription drugs they have been taking for migraine and migraine-related symptoms within a few days of beginning the program, as they have a detrimental effect on the treatment process. Pain killers, for example, destroy intestinal flora and upset the balance in the digestive system, as well as have a negative impact on various hormone levels. Fortunately, patients begin to see results from the Migraine Cure within just a few days.

Neurohormonal System

Our overview of the Migraine Cure begins with a discussion of the foundation of the treatment program, the neurohormonal system, which is a vast communication system composed of hormones, hormone messengers, hormone receptors, and nerve pathways that work together to maintain a balanced relationship among the various organs and systems it serves. A key component of the neurohormonal system is the hypothalamic-pituitary-adrenal axis, or HPA axis for short, and its relationship with the steroid hormones. Proper functioning of all the components of the HPA axis is essential for eliminating migraine. Here I have provided a simplified illustration of the HPA axis, which you can refer to during our discussion here and while reading subsequent chapters to help you visualize this process.

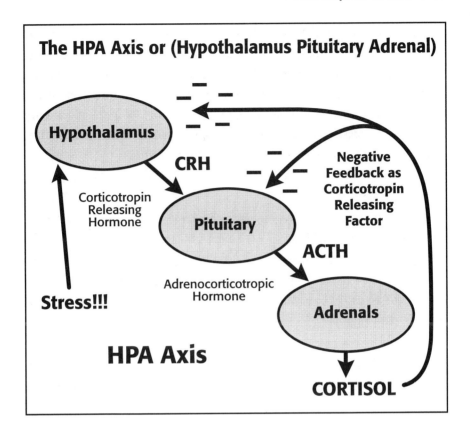

The HPA Axis or (Hypothalamus Pituitary Adrenal)

Hypothalamus

We first turn to the hypothalamus, a tiny piece of tissue deep in the brain that serves as the control center for the majority of the body's hormonal systems and is responsible for regulating homeostasis, a stable state of equilibrium. The hypothalamus takes in information from many different internal and external sources, including sensory data from what you see, taste, smell, touch, and hear; and the hormone melatonin, which is transmitted from the pineal gland (see below). The hypothalamus then embarks on various tasks.

In response to physical or psychological stress, for example, cells in the hypothalamus determine how much cortisol your body needs and produces corticotropin-releasing hormone (CRH). The CRH travels to the pituitary gland, where it binds to specific receptors on cells in the gland, which then produces adreno-corticotropic hormone (ACTH). This hormone is transported to the adrenal gland, where it stimulates the production of adrenal hormones. The adrenals increase their secretion of cortisol, and the cortisol then initiates metabolic actions aimed at alleviating the harmful effects of stress through negative feedback to the hypothalamus and the pituitary, which decreases the concentration of ACTH and cortisol in the blood once the stress subsides. The pituitary also releases beta-endorphin, a morphine-like hormone that helps reduce pain during times of stress.

The hypothalamus can influence the development and occurrence of migraine in several ways. For example, the hypothalamus:

- Helps activate the parasympathetic nervous system, which needs to be in balance with the sympathetic nervous system to eliminate migraine.

- Directly or indirectly stimulates release of certain hormones from the pituitary gland, adrenal glands, ovaries, and testes that are key players in migraine. For example:

  — Controls release of melatonin, a hormone that is effective in preventing migraine.

  — Stimulates the release of adreno-corticotropic hormone (ACTH), which in turn initiates the production of the hormone cortisol, which helps restore homeostasis after stress. The amount of cortisol in circulation is also important because it has a unique relationship with DHEA, a hormone that is critical in the development and elimination of migraine. I talk more about the DHEA-to-cortisol ratio below.

  — Indirectly has an impact on the production of estrogen and progesterone, two hormones that are key players in migraine.

Pituitary Gland

The pituitary gland is a pea-sized structure that is located at the base of the brain and is attached to the hypothalamus by nerve fibers. This tiny gland is divided into three sections, or lobes, each one of which produces certain hormones when prompted by the hypothalamus. As noted above, the pituitary gland secretes ACTH, one of the hormones produced in the anterior lobe. The ACTH leaves the pituitary gland and travels to the adrenal cortex, where it stimulates the release of the hormone cortisol, which, as noted above, is a key factor in maintaining homeostasis. Cortisol also has many other roles in the body, including the regulation of protein, fat, and carbohydrate metabolism and blood pressure.

The pituitary also releases follicle-stimulating hormone (FSH), a substance that travels to the ovaries and stimulates the development of follicles, fluid-filled sacs that contain eggs. The FSH also stimulates the secretion of estrogen (estradiol) from the follicles and has an effect on the amount of estrogen that is released into the bloodstream and thus a critical impact on the amount of estrogen that must be balanced against progesterone.

Adrenal Glands

Sitting atop each of the kidneys is an adrenal gland. These orange-colored, triangular-shaped glands are about three inches in length and are each composed of a medulla (inner part) and a cortex (outer part), which itself consists of three zones, named below. Each of the zones in the adrenal cortex contains cholesterol, and an enzyme called CYP11A then converts the cholesterol into pregnenolone, which is the first hormone produced in each of the three zones. Each zone then goes on to manufacture specific steroid hormones from the pregnenolone — all of which are important in migraine — with the help of other special enzymes.

- Zona glomerulosa produces aldosterone, a mineralocorticoid that maintains blood volume and pressure by controlling the sodium-to-potassium balance of the blood.

- Zona fasciculata produces cortisol, a stress hormone that performs many functions, including reduction in the harmful effects of stress, anti-inflammatory actions and blood sugar regulation. If the adrenal glands do not produce enough cortisol, various signs and symptoms can develop, including headache, gastrointestinal problems, fatigue, dizziness, and low blood sugar, among others.

- Zona reticularis produces progesterone, DHEA and DHEA-S, and a small amount of estrogens and testosterone, although most of these latter two hormones are produced by the ovaries and testes.

- Medulla produces adrenaline (epinephrine), which is secreted in response to signals from the hypothalamus and is a sympathetic nervous system response often referred to as "fight or flight" situations. The medulla also produces noradrenaline (norepinephrine), which helps regulate the wake-sleep cycle, among other tasks.

There is a special relationship between cortisol and DHEA, which is a precursor to the sex hormones testosterone and the estrogens. The DHEA-to-cortisol ratio increases when you are calm or in a low-stress situation but decreases during illness and acute stress. We will explore this ratio and its importance to migraine in more detail in chapter 4 on hormones.

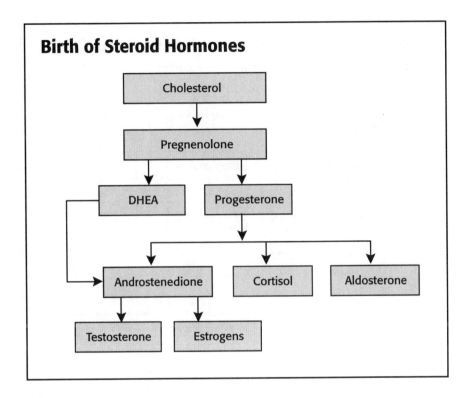

Adrenal Insufficiency

Because optimal functioning of the adrenal glands is critical for hormone production, and thus elimination of migraine, I want to talk briefly about a common condition called *adrenal insufficiency*, also known as adrenal fatigue. Adrenal insufficiency occurs when the adrenal glands are damaged or overworked, usually due to long-term or chronic stress. This type of stress can include chronic pain (e.g., migraine), chronic inflammation, chronic infections, lack of sleep, intake of excess sugar or caffeine, exposure to environmental toxins (e.g., secondhand smoke), low blood sugar, and simply the often overwhelming stress of everyday life with its high demands from work, navigating traffic, financial worries, raising children, having to care for elderly or sick parents, and often feeling as if one has to "do it all."

Adrenal insufficiency develops gradually. What happens is this: chronic stress causes the adrenals to produce large amounts of cortisol and adrenaline. At the same time, production of DHEA declines. Increased production

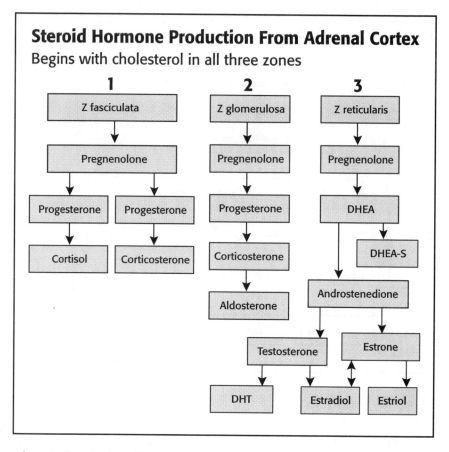

Steroid Hormone Production From Adrenal Cortex
Begins with cholesterol in all three zones

of cortisol and adrenaline continues and then drops to a normal level. The body has amazing powers of resistance, and so to make up for the reduced production of cortisol and adrenaline, a phenomenon called "pregnenolone steal" occurs, in which production of this hormone as well as DHEA, progesterone, estrogens, and testosterone (because pregnenolone is a precursor of these hormones) decline in favor of cortisol. Eventually, however, the adrenals burnout and cortisol and adrenaline levels are depleted and severe imbalances of the other steroid hormones occurs.

Symptoms of adrenal insufficiency are no stranger to many migraineurs: fatigue (especially in the morning and between 3 and 5 pm when cortisol levels decline), insomnia, reduce sex drive, reduced memory and concentration, indigestion, alternating diarrhea and constipation, anxiety, chronic pain (especially in the neck and upper back), unexplained hair loss, poor blood sugar control, and depression.

Adrenal insufficiency is often missed or ignored by conventional doctors because normal blood tests are designed to detect the severe deficiency of adrenal hormones associated with Addison's disease. Yet adrenal hormone levels in people who have adrenal insufficiency often register as "normal" even though the levels can be half of the optimum level and still be considered "normal" by most physicians and labs. Unfortunately, this misconception leads to adrenal insufficiency being missed in many individuals, especially women.

The Steroid Hormones

The steroid hormones—estrogens, progesterone, testosterone, DHEA, pregnenolone, and cortisol—belong to a family of natural hormones that are very similar in structure, yet the minute differences among them are responsible for some very significant differences in how they function. The predominantly female hormone estrogen, for example, stimulates the development of breasts in women, while the predominantly male hormone testosterone causes facial hair growth.

So far you've seen how the activities of the components of the HPA axis lead to production of the steroid hormones. If you look at the two illustrations in this chapter (the "HPA Axis" and "Birth of Steroid Hormones") you can see that there are many steps in this production process, which means there are many factors we must consider as we attempt to restore these hormones to optimal levels. Also keep in mind that the ovaries and testes also produce steroid hormones, so the health and hormone production of these glands need to be watched as well. A deficiency or imbalance among any of the substances or processes mentioned can have a significant impact on how we treat a patient and meet our goals.

FIVE MAJOR CLASSES OF STEROID HORMONES

- Progestagens, of which progesterone is the main hormone. Progesterone is primarily a female hormone, but males have this hormone as well, albeit at low levels. In both men and women one of its primary functions is to balance or offset the effects of estrogen. It is produced primarily by the corpus luteum (an indirect product of the ovaries) in women and by the adrenals and testes in men.
- Glucocorticoids, the antistress hormones, which include cortisol and cortisone.
- Mineralcorticoids, which includes aldosterone and which functions to regulate sodium and potassium levels.
- Androgens, the male sex hormones, of which testosterone is the main hormone. In men, testosterone is responsible for, among other things, development of the male reproductive structures, increased muscular and skeletal growth, growth and distribution of body hair, and increased male sex drive. Women also have low levels of this hormone.
- Estrogen, one of the main female sex hormones, of which the three most important types are estradiol, estriol, and estrone. Males also have estrogen, but at low levels. The importance of estrogen in female physiology is supported by the fact that females have more than 300 different kinds of receptors that can be activated by the hormone, which means estrogen can have an impact of numerous functions in a woman's body.

Although we will talk about each of the hormones in depth in chapter 4, here I want to explain the relationship among them and how they relate to the components in the other two steps of the Migraine Cure. The first tests we do when we implement the Migraine Cure are the female (or male) hormone panel, which tells us the patient's steroid hormone levels, and a blood lipid panel to determine cholesterol levels. **The restoration program**

cannot proceed until we have these figures. Only then can we work toward identifying and achieving the optimal range of each hormone for the patient. Nearly every patient with migraine has deficiencies of these steroid hormones before they begin hormone restoration therapy (with notable exceptions, like Melissa above), with deficiencies in pregnenolone being the most prominent. Even in rare cases like Melissa's above, in which her hormone levels fell within "normal" ranges, we discovered that a healthy, optimal level of testosterone for Melissa was somewhat outside what was considered "normal" in the general population.

"Normal" and "Optimal" Ranges

To give you an idea of what is considered "normal" for our purposes, I have included a table that lists these hormones and two sets of figures: the "reference range" and the "optimal range" for each. These terms are important and I use them throughout the book, so let me explain what they mean.

A reference range is a set of values used by conventional medical professionals to interpret test results. The range is usually defined as values that 95 percent of the normal population falls within. Reference ranges vary, depending on the age, race, and sex of the population, as well as the instruments that perform the tests. One main problem with reference ranges is that they represent the "average" person who, in today's society, is more likely to be overweight, overstressed, and inadequately nourished than not. Another problem is that the ranges are too broad to be helpful in identifying health problems or recommending treatment for individual patients.

Another problem with reference ranges is that they are age specific. For example, a fifty-year-old woman who has migraine, fatigue, and insomnia goes to her doctor and has her hormone levels checked. The doctor announces that all her hormone levels fall within the ranges that are "normal" for her age. Unfortunately, "normal" for her age is typically far from what is optimal for her health. And *optimal* ranges are what we try to restore for people who have migraine.

For our purposes, when we talk about optimal ranges of hormone levels we are referring to levels seen in healthy 20- to 30-year-old men and women and levels required to maintain that good health. Thus when we talk about hormone restoration in this and subsequent chapters, we are talking about restoring an individual's hormone levels to this optimal range. Naturally, we need to be flexible when we consider what is optimal for each patient within each range, because every individual functions best at levels that are unique to him or her. This certainly was the case with Melissa, who functioned best when her testosterone levels were somewhat higher than seen in the "normal" population. Thus both reference ranges and optimal ranges should be viewed as guidelines only, not as absolute levels to be achieved.

In some studies, for example, migraine patients had significantly reduced levels of testosterone and significantly increased levels of cortisol, but this did not hold true for yet another study, in which testosterone levels of migraine patients were normal. Thus "normal" is a relative term, and what is optimal is unique for each patient. In our work, we found that all basic hormones must be at or close to optimal in order to eliminate migraine.

Bio-identical versus Synthetic

Another critical characteristic of the hormone restoration portion of the Migraine Cure is that all of the hormones administered are chemically identical to the hormones that the human body produces naturally. **No synthetic or biochemically unfriendly hormones are used.** When it comes to estrogen, for example, the most popular prescription in the United States is a horse-urine-derived product (Premarin) that is not biocompatible with the human body's naturally produced estrogen. Similarly, bio-identical progesterone is used in favor of the synthetic steroid hormones, medroxyprogesterone acetate and methyl testosterone. As you'll see in chapter 3 in our discussion of why current therapies don't work, use of these synthetic steroid hormones is not only ineffective but medically hazardous as well.

Another feature of the program is that the hormones are given in doses and according to a schedule that simulate the patient's natural human hormone production and cycles. That means, for example, women receive doses of estrogens and progesterone that mimic their natural monthly hormonal cycle. A balance between these two hormones also contributes to a balance between the sympathetic and parasympathetic systems, because estrogen stimulates the sympathetic system while progesterone affects the parasympathetic.

	Reference Range	Optimal Range
Total cholesterol	<200 mg/dL	170-200 mg/dL
Total estrogen (females only)	61-437 pg/mL	250-437 pg/mL
Estradiol (males only)	0-53 pg/mL	<25 pg/mL
Progesterone		
Females	0.2-28 ng/mL	6-28 ng/mL
Males	0.3-1.2 ng/mL	1-1.2 ng/mL
Total testosterone		
Females	14-76 ng/dL	60-76 ng/dL
Males	241-827 ng/dL	650-827 ng/dL
DHEA-S		
Females	65-380 ug/dL	250-380 ug/dL
Males	280-640 ug/dL	500-640 ug/dL
Pregnenolone		
Females	10-230 ng/dL	200-230 ng/dL
Males	10-200 ng/dL	180-200 ng/dL
Cortisol (a.m.)	4.3-22.4 ug/dL	15-22.4 ug/dL

Pineal Gland

The pineal gland is a pine cone-shaped structure (thus its name) located deep in the brain. It is activated by light which it receives via a complex route originating in the eye and works closely with the hypothalamus to help control various biorhythms. Its primary function is to produce and secrete melatonin, a hormone that is associated with the sleep-wake circadian (daily) cycle. Research has shown that dysfunction of the pineal gland can result in a deficiency of melatonin, which has been shown to cause migraine. Similarly, supplementation of melatonin to migraine patients can result in pain relief and a reduction in the recurrence of head pain. Therefore I believe that ensuring the healthy function of the pineal gland is critical for elimination of migraine. I explore this relationship in detail in chapter 5.

Digestive System

It's a generally recognized fact that if the gastrointestinal tract, or gut, is not functioning in a healthy manner, the rest of the body can't be healthy either. This relationship becomes clearer when we consider the tasks of the gut. Basically, the gut:

- Digests food
- Absorbs food elements, which are then converted into energy
- Transports nutrients out of the gut into the bloodstream so they can be utilized by the body
- Plays a major role in ridding the body of toxins that can cause or contribute to a wide range of medical problems, including migraine
- Contains substances that are the body's first line of defense against infection

Restoring and maintaining the health and integrity of the gut is all too often overlooked by physicians, regardless of the condition they are treating. Many of the components and their functions in the gut have direct and significant links with the development of migraine as well as other components of the program, and so achieving a healthy gut is absolutely essential for elimination of migraine.

This step of the Migraine Cure focuses primarily on:

- Restoring healthy intestinal flora through supplementation with friendly bacteria, or probiotics. I discuss the importance of a balanced intestinal flora in chapter 5, but here I want to mention that such a balance is essential to adequately absorb nutrients and avoid toxic reactions, including migraine, inflammatory disorders, gas, diarrhea, constipation, eczema, fatigue, and other signs and symptoms of an imbalance between the sympathetic and parasympathetic nervous systems. For example, most people who have migraine also suffer with constipation, which is a reflection of abnormal intestinal flora but also dominance of the sympathetic nervous system. Irritable bowel syndrome, also seen among migraineurs, is a reflection of an imbalance between the sympathetic and parasympathetic systems as well.

- Maintaining a proper balance between calcium, which stimulates the sympathetic nervous system; and magnesium, which stimulates the parasympathetic system. When these two minerals are out of balance, there are serious changes in the cell membranes which affect the electrical stability of the cells and their sensitivity to messages from the steroid hormones, melatonin, and serotonin.

Serotonin

Why are we talking about serotonin in the digestive system? Isn't serotonin found mainly in the brain? Although the pineal gland is the richest site of serotonin in the brain, only about 5 percent of the serotonin in the body is found in the brain. Ninety-five percent resides in the gastrointestinal tract, where it plays a major role in modulating the perception of pain and regulating secretions and movement in the intestinal tract, which helps the digestive system operate normally. We know, for example, that when certain receptors in the gut's lining are stimulated, serotonin is released, which triggers peristalsis.

Recent studies show that some gastrointestinal disorders are related to an imbalance of serotonin in the gut, an abnormal reaction of the digestive system to serotonin, or faulty communication between serotonin in the gut and the brain and spinal cord. Thus abnormal serotonin levels have been linked to many health problems, including migraine, cluster headache, and depression (low serotonin levels) and anorexia, bulimia, and anxiety (high levels). Thus once again here is another substance that has an impact in more than one system in this migraine complex, and we need to restore and maintain a balance among these substances if we are to eliminate migraine. We'll further explore the relationship between serotonin, the gut, and migraine in chapter 6.

Sympathetic and Parasympathetic Nervous Systems

I have emphasized that the basis of the Migraine Cure is a balance between the sympathetic and parasympathetic nervous systems, which is achieved when as we restore balance to the other components of the program. But because the terms "sympathetic" and "parasympathetic" are alien to most people, and because the vital roles they play in migraine are a mystery to the majority of people as well, some explanation is in order. That explanation begins with its parent system, the autonomic nervous system.

The Autonomic Nervous System

The organs of your body, such as your heart, intestines, stomach, and bladder, are regulated by a part of the central nervous system (which is composed of the brain and spinal cord) called the autonomic nervous system (ANS). More specifically, the ANS controls the muscles of these organs, as well as the muscles in the skin, the eye, and the blood vessels, and also works with the endocrine system to control the secretion of hormones. It does all this by conveying sensory signals from the various organs and glands through nerves to parts of the brain, mainly the hypothalamus (remember the hypothalamus from our discussion of the neurohormonal system), medulla, and pons.

The Sympathetic and Parasympathetic Nervous Systems

The ANS is composed of three subgroups, two of which are of special importance to our discussion of migraine; namely, the sympathetic and parasympathetic nervous systems. Both of these systems operate continuously and simultaneously but in varying degrees. The ANS provides nearly every organ with a double set of nerves—one sympathetic and one parasympathetic. Thus both systems are always having an impact on the same organs, but their impact differs both in degree and in effect. For instance, when a stressful situation arises, the actions of the sympathetic nervous system dominate, but once the situation changes and the stress is reduced or eliminated, the parasympathetic system will dominate and cause an opposite effect and bring the body back to a state of equilibrium or homeostasis. You can liken it to operating your car: you use your brakes to slow down and your accelerator to speed up, and you balance the two to give you a balanced (within the speed limit!) ride. Thus the actions of one nervous system balance the actions of the other and restore (or attempt to restore) harmony.

What does any of this have to do with migraine? Plenty. Our research has shown us that migraine is the result of an imbalance among several critical systems in the body, and the culmination of those imbalances are reflected in the sympathetic and parasympathetic nervous systems. Thus when we balance the components of the individual systems, we restore balance to these two complementary nervous systems. An imbalance between these two systems also leads to a reduction in the pain threshold of the brain's nociceptive system. This system controls nociceptive pain, which is caused when specific nerve endings, called nociceptors, are irritated. Nociceptive pain can be mild or severe, acute or chronic, and is characterized by a sharp or dull aching pain, such as when you twist your ankle or stub your toe, or the pain associated with arthritis or cancer.

The Balancing Act at Work

Here's an example of how this balancing act works. The sympathetic nervous system is an energy user and is known as the "fight or flight" system, because it springs into action in stressful situations. Say, for example, you and your six-year-old daughter are walking through a parking lot after finishing lunch at a pizza restaurant. Suddenly she breaks free of your hand and steps into the path of an oncoming car. Immediately you rush toward her to save her.

At the same time, your sympathetic nervous system bursts into action, raising your heart rate and increasing your blood pressure and blood flow away from your periphery and digestive system and toward your brain, heart, and skeletal muscles, which are where you need your energy to be focused at that time. You also experience a dramatic increase in the amount of adrenaline in your blood stream, which temporarily increases your physical strength. You use that strength to pull your daughter back safely into your arms.

The stressful situation is now over, and so your parasympathetic nervous system takes over: your heart beat gradually returns to normal, your blood pressure decreases, the level of adrenaline declines, and your stomach resumes digesting the pizza you had for lunch.

Of course, most of the stressors in your life are not so dramatic, yet the sympathetic and parasympathetic systems are still hard at work, with one dominating and then the other, twenty-four hours a day. Emotional stress, for example, can raise blood pressure and pump high amounts of stress hormones (e.g., cortisol) into your blood stream. The stress of poor dietary habits can cause deficiencies of serotonin and melatonin, and low levels of melatonin are associated with migraine. Similarly, an imbalance in the ratio of magnesium to calcium is associated with migraine. These and many other stressors can cause an imbalance between these two nervous systems, stressors that have a significant impact on the development of migraine. We will explore these stressors in detail in this chapter and in the chapters on hormones, the pineal gland, and the digestive system, and show you how to restore balance among them.

Are You Talking To Me?

I have already described the neurohormonal system as a vast communication network, and so, too, are the sympathetic and parasympathetic nervous systems. Both of these systems have elements that communicate not only with each other but also with components in other systems as well, such as the digestive system and the pineal gland, key factors in the Migraine Cure. This entire communication network is very complex and would take volumes to explain, but there are a few things you should know.

To assist with the communication between the sympathetic and parasympathetic systems, the ANS provides each of the organs with a double set of nerves, one sympathetic and one parasympathetic. Messages (nerve impulses) are carried along these nerves with the help of chemical substances called neurotransmitters, such as acetylcholine, norepinephrine, and serotonin. To help convey messages, the sympathetic system uses both

OPPOSING ACTIONS OF THE SYMPATHETIC AND PARASYMPATHETIC NERVOUS SYSTEMS

When these specific areas of the body are stimulated by either the sympathetic or parasympathetic nervous system, the following responses may occur:

	Sympathetic	Parasympathetic
Iris	Pupils dilate	Pupils constrict
Heart	Rate and force increase	Rate and force decrease
Kidney	Decreased urine production	Increased urine production
Lungs	Bronchi dilate	Bronchi constrict
Salivary glands	Saliva production decreases	Saliva production increases
Oral/nasal mucosa	Mucus production decreases	Mucus production increases
Sweat glands	Secrete sweat	No secretion
Gastrointestinal	Constipation, intestines relax, peristalsis and tone decrease	Nausea, vomiting, diarrhea, gastric juice secretions increase, peristalsis increases, sphincters relax

acetylcholine and norepinephrine. The acetylcholine affects calcium ions, sodium, and potassium, which is important in the development and elimination of migraine, while norepinephrine impacts the sympathetic nervous system (except for sweat glands). The parasympathetic nervous system also uses acetylcholine, but in this system it innervates the smooth muscles of organs and prompts them into action.

In Conclusion

Migraine is a complex syndrome with multiple causes and multiple components that then interact with each other in ways that can work to either cause or prevent migraine and its associated symptoms. If you would like to participate in the Migraine Cure program, contact Dr. Sergey Dzugan and his medical staff at 1-877-402-2721 or at www.fountain-migraine.com; or contact The Life Extension Foundation, 1-800-226-2370; www.lef.org.

In this chapter I introduced the four primary systems that contribute to migraine and how the Migraine Cure addresses those components to bring about balance between the sympathetic and parasympathetic nervous systems and eliminate migraine. We will explore each of those systems in detail and the Migraine Cure in its entirety in future chapters. First, however, let's look at the treatments that are currently being prescribed to treat migraine and why they don't work.

3

Why Current Therapies Don't Work

Katherine, a thirty-eight-year-old software engineer, had just left the office of Dr. W, the fifth and, she said, last doctor she was going to see about her migraines. "I've had it to here," she said, drawing a line with her hand above her head. "Every doctor tells me the same thing: 'avoid stress, avoid certain foods and other things that trigger the pain, and keep taking the medications.' But I do all that, and it doesn't work. I still get two or three migraines a month. I miss work, I miss time with my family, and I miss my life."

Katherine's story could be yours and the story of millions of other women and men who suffer with migraine and who are looking for relief. When you look around, there is relief, lots of it, in the form of prescription and over-the-counter medications, herbal remedies, stress reduction methods, body work therapies, nutritional supplements, energy therapies, and psychological interventions. Each and every one of these treatment approaches can provide some level of symptom relief for a limited amount of time, but the unfortunate truth is that **these current therapies don't work because none of them addresses the root causes of migraine.** Using these various treatment methods is like repeatedly applying small adhesive bandages to a gaping wound: you can keep putting them on, but they are ineffective and keep falling off. They don't stick. The Migraine Cure "sticks" because it addresses the causes of migraine.

To make matters worse, migraineurs generally are very dissatisfied with the current treatment options not only because they aren't effective but also because they are often accompanied by adverse effects. It is generally accepted, for example, that about 35 percent of patients who take sumatriptan—the most commonly prescribed medication for migraine—and similar migraine medications will experience another migraine attack within 24 hours of treatment. And one look at the side effects that are associated with the arsenal of drugs used to treat migraine is enough to make anyone think twice about taking them (see Table later in this chapter).

When it comes to side effects, in one study researchers found that 44.5 percent of the patients reported adverse events—including dizziness, headache, nausea, difficulty in thinking, fatigue, and tingling of the toes and fingers — after using various medications. Some patients are so discouraged by the side effects that they elect to forego treatment rather than suffer additional pain and discomfort.

If current therapies don't work, why should we bother looking at them? Several reasons. One, because some of them offer insight into why the steps we take in the Migraine Cure do work. Two, because some of these therapies are good for your health, and it would be a good idea to incorporate them into your lifestyle. Stress management techniques such as visualization and progressive relaxation, for example, can be very beneficial for overall physical, mental, emotional, and spiritual well-being.

Needed: An Attitude Adjustment

As if the lack of effective migraine treatments is not enough, migraineurs also have to contend with widespread myths and bad attitudes. Although migraine clearly is a physiological disease, some health-care practitioners still believe that migraine is a condition that an individual must "learn to live with" or that stress is the main cause of migraine. Some even go so far as to suggest that it's "all in your head." Practitioners who persist in their belief that migraine is a psychological disorder often tell patients that they are clinically depressed and that they need antidepressants or other medications typically prescribed to treat depression. Generally these drugs are not helpful and may even be detrimental. Although many people with migraine do suffer with depression as part of the disease of migraine, doctors' failure to recognize and treat migraine as a distinct medical entity leaves many patients both misdiagnosed and treated ineffectively, if at all, and many become frustrated with the medical community and just try to treat themselves the best way they can.

Problems With Conventional Hormone Replacement Therapy

It's well-known that migraine affects approximately three times as many women as men and that in many women a menstrual-related migraine occurs when the levels of estrogen decline before and during the first day or two of menstruation. In fact, migraines occur during menstruation in about 60 percent of women migraineurs. On a positive note, research also indicates that most pregnant women who have menstrual or non-menstrual migraines before they get pregnant are either migraine-free or experience an improvement in their migraines during pregnancy, and that the improvement is more significant for women who had menstrual migraines than those who did not.

These findings lead some researchers to posit that the administration of hormone replacement therapy or birth control pills could be used to treat menstrual-related migraine. This way of thinking is close to the mark, and countless numbers of women follow—and continue to follow — this treatment approach, even though it is not terribly effective. According to the British Migraine Association, hormone replacement therapy results in an improvement in migraine frequency in 45 percent, worsens it in 46 percent, and leaves it unchanged in 9 percent.

But there is an even darker cloud over the practice of conventional hormone replacement therapy, and it is one which, as it turns out, was probably a good thing because it focused attention on a practice that was on the right track, but not close enough. Here's what happened.

First, a little refresher. To treat symptoms such as night sweats, hot flashes, vaginal dryness, mood swings, and breast tenderness that often develop as women approach menopause, doctors often prescribe hormone therapy. Because estrogen taken alone stimulates tissue growth, and thus increases the risk of cancer in areas such as the breast and uterus, women who have an intact uterus are usually advised to take synthetic progestin along with the estrogen to suppress this type of growth. In other words, the addition of progesterone is supposed to balance or offset the effects of estrogen. This type of therapy is known as hormone replacement therapy (HRT).

Perhaps you remember the landmark Women's Health Initiative study in which women were given hormone replacement therapy in the form of Prempro, a drug that contains a combination of synthetic estrogen and progestin in a single daily pill. The study was conducted with 16,608 women ages 50 to 79 who had an intact uterus and was scheduled to run until 2005. It was halted in July 2002 when the researchers realized that the participants who were taking the hormones showed an increased risk of heart attack (increased risk, 29%), total cardiovascular disease (22%), and breast cancer (26%) when compared with women who were taking a placebo. The discovery scared many women and caused a great number of them across the country to discontinue hormone therapy.

I and some of my colleagues had already recognized that the WHI study was problematic, for reasons that I discuss below. Conventional medicine was reluctant initially to point out the study's flaws, but it was only a matter of time before they came to light. One of the more recent articles was published in December 2005 in *Fertility and Sterility* by Edward Klaiber, MD, an endocrinologist, and his colleagues, who concluded that the study and the results were basically flawed, that "Prempro was a mistake," and that "the results might have been different if they had used a different form of estrogen that resembled a normal cycle."

Other experts, like DG Stein, PhD, at Emory University School of Medicine, commented on clinical trials that used synthetic hormones and argued in the *Annals of New York Academy of Science* that "the data do not reflect what might have been the case if [natural estrogen] had been tested with natural progesterone instead of synthetic medroxyprogesterone acetate."

What the WHI succeeded in doing was throwing out the baby with the bath water: it frightened women away from a therapeutic approach that can be very effective **if it is administered properly,** as we do in the Migraine Cure.

WHAT'S WRONG WITH CONVENTIONAL HORMONE REPLACEMENT THERAPY?

Here's a brief rundown:

- Physicians often prescribe hormones that are not bio-identical to those naturally produced in the human body, therefore they do not function nor contribute to the operation of other functions the way they should.

- Even if physicians prescribe hormones that are bio-identical, all three of the necessary estrogens are not available as patented hormones. Estriol, for example, is not currently available as a patented estrogen drug, although you can get it at a compounding pharmacy with a doctor's prescription. Thus unless your doctor writes a prescription for the correct balance of the three estrogens in a bio-identical form, you will not achieve your optimal balance of this hormone.

- Hormones are typically prescribed without evaluating a woman's hormone levels before treatment and without monitoring hormone levels during treatment. In fact, it is not unusual for doctors and their patients to have no idea what a woman's estrogen and progesterone levels are.

- Hormones are not administered according to each woman's specific physiological requirements. Because estrogen and progesterone levels change daily, doses of these hormones should be tailored to meet each woman's hormonal cycle. However, because the synthetic hormones that have been approved by the Food and Drug Administration (FDA) come in a one-size-fits-all formulation—a fixed dose that does not take individual differences into consideration. Thus some women are given estrogen alone for two weeks followed by an estrogen/progestin combination for the second two weeks, while others take a combination drug for the entire month.

> • Failure to address the imbalance of other hormones associated with migraine, including testosterone, pregnenolone, and DHEA. This is an area most doctors ignore completely, but I have found that it is critical to balance these hormones along with estrogen and progesterone to not only eliminate migraine, but rid the body of other serious medical conditions as well (see chapter 9).

The result of using conventional hormone therapy is a continued imbalance of hormones, failure to eliminate migraine, and the possibility of placing women at higher risk of serious medical conditions, such as stroke, heart attack, osteoporosis, Alzheimer's disease, and various cancers, among other problems.

My research shows that not only is it critical to achieve a balance between these hormones, but the supplements used to restore those hormones **must** be bio-identical to be effective. This is important for several reasons. One, to eliminate migraine you need to use biocompatible hormones to allow the body to achieve a natural balance. Two, synthetic hormones are foreign to the body and are associated with significant health risks. Many studies have suggested, for example, that the addition of progestins (the term for synthetic progesterone) to estrogen in hormone replacement therapy increases a woman's risk of breast cancer when compared to estrogen alone, whereas a recent study indicates that adding natural progesterone to such treatment does not affect breast cancer risk. Some women who take progestins to alleviate symptoms of PMS or to oppose estrogen in menopause experience mood swings, bloating, and headache when they take this synthetic hormone. Those who take natural micronized progesterone, however, report that their mood swings, fluid retention, and headaches are completely or mostly eliminated. Clearly, bio-identical is the way to go.

Problems With Drugs

"I can't believe that the very drugs I was given to relieve my symptoms are actually causing migraines." This statement from a very frustrated migraineur echoes the experiences of many migraine patients and is just one of the problems with the use of drugs to treat this disease. Indeed, the use of beta blockers, calcium channel blockers, ergots, and even some over-the-counter non-narcotic painkillers can trigger migraines if they are used consistently. But this is not the only problem with medications.

"I never imagined that the quality of my life would depend on drugs, but it does," says Brigette, a thirty-eight-year-old fashion designer who lives in New York City. "I need drugs every day to help prevent a migraine attack, other drugs when I feel an attack coming on, and still more drugs if the other ones haven't done the job. Then there are the drugs I could take to treat the other symptoms that come with migraine, like constipation and insomnia. But I try to avoid them because there are side effects, and it just gets too complicated. I've been getting one or two migraines a month for more than ten years, and I'm tired of being sick and tired."

Bridgett's story is not unusual. Millions of migraineurs depend on drugs to help them get through the day. The drugs at their disposal fall into two general categories: those prescribed to prevent migraine (referred to as pro-phylactic drugs) and those that attempt to stop symptoms as they are starting and/or to treat active migraine symptoms. There are a sizeable number of drugs in each category, and subgroups within each, which you can see in the accompanying table. Let's look at the two categories and how they work... or don't work.

Prophylactic Drugs

According to the American College of Physicians and the American Society of Internal Medicine, prophylactic medications are suggested for migraine patients if they meet at least one of the following criteria: two or more migraine attacks per month that produce disability that lasts three days or longer; failure to respond to or an inability to take other migraine medications; need to use abortive medications more than twice a week;

and/or presence of uncommon migraine, such as migraine with a prolonged aura or hemiplegic migraine. You must take prophylactic medications every day, and it usually takes two to six weeks before you will know whether any specific drug will help you. The chance that a given drug will be effective is 50 to 75 percent, and it is not unusual for patients to try three or more drugs before they find one that provides some relief. Drugs in this category include nonsteroid anti-inflammatory drugs (NSAIDs), tricyclic antidepressants, selective serotonin reuptake inhibitors (a type of antidepressant), anticonvulsants, beta-blockers, and calcium channel blockers.

PREVENTIVE DRUG TREATMENT

DRUG	SIDE EFFECTS
Anticonvulsants	
Divalproex (Depakene)	Diarrhea, stomach cramps, hair loss, nausea, vomiting, hand trembling
Gabapentin (Neurontin	Clumsiness, uncontrolled eye movements
Topiramate (Topamax)	Drowsiness, weight gain, tingling in arms, nausea
Valproic acid (Depakote)	Nausea, drowsiness, weight gain, tremors
Antidepressants (Tricyclics)	
Amitriptyline (Elavil)	Generally, all tricyclics can cause
Desipramine (Norpramin)	dizziness, dry mouth, drowsiness,
Doxepin (Sinequan)	headache, nausea, weight gain,
Imipramine (Tofranil)	weakness
Nortriptyline (Pamelor)	
Antidepressants (SSRIs)	
Fluoxetine (Prozac)	Nausea, dry mouth, increased appetite, agitation
Paroxetine (Paxil)	Fatigue, weight gain
Sertraline (Zoloft)	Insomnia, restlessness
Venlafaxine (Effexor)	Vision problems, sexual decline, headache

Antidepressants (Other)

Bupropion (Wellbutrin)

Agitation, anxiety, rash, itching, ringing ears

Trazodone (Deseryl)

Dizziness, drowsiness, dry mouth, headache, nausea, vomiting, unpleasant taste

Beta-Blockers

Atenolol (Tenormin)

All beta-blockers can cause depression, memory disturbances, diarrhea, faintness, weight gain

Metoprolol (Lopressor)
Nadolol (Corgard)
Propranolol (Inderal)
Timolol (Blocadren)

Calcium-Channel Blockers

Amlodipine

Diltiazem (Cardizem)

Dizziness, constipation

Nicardipine (Cardene)

Drowsiness, increased appetite, weight gain

Nifedipine (Procardia)

Drowsiness, increased appetite, weight gain

Nimodipine (Nimotop)

Drowsiness, increased appetite, weight gain

Verapamil (Calan, Isoptin)

Constipation, dizziness

NSAIDS

Celecoxib (Celebrex)

Diclofenac (Cataflam)

Stomach upset, dizziness, drowsiness

Fenoprofen (Lodine)

GI upset, drowsiness, dizziness, vision problems, ulcers

Ibuprofen (Haltran, Medipren, Motrin, Q-Profen)

GI upset, drowsiness, dizziness, vision problems, ulcers

Ketaprofen (Actron, Orudis)

GI upset, nausea, vomiting, rash, liver damage

Naproxen (Aleve, Anaprox)

GI upset, nausea, vomiting, rash, liver damage

Serotonin Agonist

Methyseride

ABORTIVE, AND SYMPTOMATIC DRUG TREATMENT

DRUG	SIDE EFFECTS
Over-the-Counter	
Acetaminophen-caffeine (Excedrin Migraine, Excedrin)	Anxiety, heartburn, insomnia, liver damage, dizziness, bruising easily
Aspirin	GI bleeding
Diclofenac (Cataflam)	See above
Ibuprofen (Motrin)	See above
Ketorolac (Toradol)	GI upset, drowsiness, dizziness, vision problems, ulcers
Meclofenamate (Meclomen)	GI upset, drowsiness, dizziness, vision problems, ulcers
Naproxen (Aleve)	See above
Ergots	
Dihydroergotamine (DHE-45, Migranal intranasal)	Nausea, numbness of fingers and toes
Ergotamine tartrate (Cafergot)	Nausea, cramps, agitation
Ergotamine (Bellergal)	drowsiness, blurry vision, dry mouth
Vasoconstrictor Combo	
Acetaminophen, isometheptene and dichlor- alphenazone (Midrin Duradrin)	Nausea, sedation
Serotonin Receptor Agonists	
Almotriptan (Axert)	All triptans have similar side effects,
Eletriptan (Relpax)	including head, jaw, chest, and arm
Flovatriptan (Frova)	discomfort, tightening, or tingling;
Naratriptan (Amerge)	throat discomfort, muscle cramps,
Rizatriptan (Maxalt)	flushing
Sumatriptan (Imitrex)	
Zolmitriptan (Zomig)	

Drugs to Abort Migraine or Treat Active Symptoms

Drugs in this category include over-the-counter and prescription medications, such as the NSAIDs ibuprofen and naproxen; the ergot drugs; vasoconstriction combination drugs; and serotonin receptor agonists, also known as triptans, of which the most commonly prescribed is sumatriptan (Imitrex®). Both ergot drugs and triptans influence serotonin levels, while NSAIDs and vasoconstriction drugs impact inflammation. One major problem with repeated use of over-the-counter painkillers is that they can reduce serotonin levels in the body, which can result in rebound headache—head pain that results from taking too many painkillers.

Important Thoughts About Other Migraine Therapies

I have already established that the reason conventional and alternative therapies for migraine don't cure migraine is because they don't address the core causes of migraine. Drug therapy and conventional hormone replacement therapy are the two biggest offenders.

Migraineurs often turn to a wide variety of other therapies as well, and they, too, do not provide lasting relief. These include, among others, acupuncture, biofeedback, chiropractic, herbal remedies such as feverfew and valerian, nutritional therapy, elimination diets, and an array of relaxation and stress-reduction techniques, including meditation, massage, visualization, progressive relaxation, guided imagery, and exercise.

Please don't misunderstand me: I am not saying that these techniques are without merit. In fact, I encourage people who have participated in the Migraine Cure to adopt healthy eating and sleeping habits, and to incorporate stress-reduction practices into their lifestyle. But I also firmly believe that it is impossible to control stress on a permanent basis unless and until hormonal balance is restored. Therefore,

You must first rid yourself of migraine.

Once you have accomplished that goal, then you are ready to live life to the fullest. Many former migraineurs had to deny themselves of so much in life or restrict their activities that they need time to revel in their new-found or restored freedoms. Suddenly, they can eat foods they could not even dream of eating when they suffered with migraine or go places they used to avoid. "I can eat chocolate and oranges again," says one former migraineur. "And I don't have to avoid places that have bright overhead lights or worry every time the barometric pressure drops. All of those things used to trigger migraines for me. But not anymore."

Some former migraineurs are anxious to try new hobbies or join new groups; others are eager to return to the life they had before the migraines started, or want to restore order to the life they had been living. "I want to travel," says Becky, who had migraines for eleven years. "I couldn't take the chance when I was getting a migraine about twice a month. But now, I've already booked a cruise, and I'm planning to fly to Europe next year." Doris, a fifty-six-year-old former editor, says she's just so grateful that now she can play with her grandchildren, take them to the zoo and shopping, and not have to worry about getting a migraine or experiencing the over-whelming fatigue she used to feel. Roger, a thirty-eight-year-old construc-tion worker, says he plans to "drink more beer and go to more parties," while forty-three-year-old Carly says she's going to "take up jogging, to keep up with my boyfriend. I might even lose some weight!"

Basically, every former migraineur is a unique individual, and once migraine is no longer a part of their lives, some people will make small changes and others will make significant ones. If some of those changes include healthier eating habits, routine exercise, yoga or tai chi classes, or daily meditation, these are positive steps I do encourage. In fact, I include some suggestions regarding nutrition and stress reduction throughout the following chapters. But if people choose to not include such changes in their lives, they will still remain migraine-free as long as they maintain the balance that is achievable when they follow the migraine program discussed in this book.

Are You Ready To Be Pain Free?

Alexis had suffered with migraines for more than a decade. At least once a week, and sometimes twice, she would be completely sidelined with the pain, and she would stay in a quiet, darkened room for 24 hours or more until she could face the world again. She missed family outings, friends' birthday parties, shopping trips, and seeing her children in school plays. She couldn't plan to go on any trips that didn't make allowances for her to "hide out" when a migraine hit. Plane travel was impossible; making long-range plans was out as well.

So when Alexis learned about the Migraine Cure, Tom, her husband, thought she would be anxious to try it, and he said he would do whatever he could to help. Yet once Alexis got all the information and spoke with others who had become migraine-free on the program, she didn't move forward with treatment. When Tom asked her what was wrong, she said she just didn't know if she could do it, but would not explain herself any further. Tom didn't understand her reluctance. Didn't she want to rid herself of this debilitating condition? Didn't she want to have a chance to participate in all the things she had missed for so many years?

Yes, and no. Alexis, like some people who have other debilitating and/or serious medical conditions, derive some benefits, or "secondary gain" from having their ailments. Migraine is painful, but it is reliable, even predictable, whereas the unknown or the unfamiliar can be frightening. As the saying goes: "Better the devil you know than the devil you don't." For other people, having migraine attacks allows them to avoid various people, situations, and obligations—some pleasant but some not so pleasant—for years, perhaps decades.

Julie, who has a sister who suffers with migraine, likened it to smoking. Although Julie was fully aware of all the health dangers, she explains that she smoked nearly three packs a day for more than eight years. One day she came down with a bad case of the flu, and she couldn't tolerate smoke for a few days. That's when Julie decided to quit cold turkey. During her withdrawal from cigarettes she experienced severe cravings, her hands trembled, and she had coughing fits. But even worse, Julie said, was that she suddenly felt frightened and confused. She explains:

"I was used to smoking all the time: while I drove, when I was on the telephone, when I was cooking, after I ate, even while I was in the shower. The first thing I did in the morning was light up a cigarette. So when I quit, I felt like I was incapable of doing all of those things. Smoking had become part of who I was, crazy as that sounds. When I got behind the wheel of the car, I couldn't even put the key into the ignition. I felt like I had forgotten how to do the simplest things. I shook when I got on the telephone and panicked when I got up in the morning because I didn't have a cigarette to turn to. My entire life changed just because I had quit smoking. And it was very scary."

Alexis eventually did follow the Migraine Cure to the letter, and now she enjoys a migraine-free life. But before she could "get with the program," she had to let go of the idea that migraine was part of who she was. Once she realized she could have the power to control migraine and that it didn't have to control her any longer, she was ready to begin the program.

In Conclusion

Every year, millions of people shell out thousands of dollars, ingest and inject various drugs, try different conventional and alternative therapies, and spend countless hours trying to prevent and treat their migraine symptoms, and unfortunately, much of their efforts are, ultimately, in vain. The migraine returns, if not that day, then the next day, or next week, or next month. Along with all their attempts there is often a feeling of frustration, anger, helplessness, and hopelessness. You know the story.

But it doesn't have to be that way. This does not have to be your story or that of anyone who has migraine. Conventional migraine treatments don't work. The Migraine Cure does. In the next four chapters we look at how it works, and how it can work for you. It's time to write your own story.

4

At Home With Your Hormones

The linchpin of the Migraine Cure can be presented in one simple statement: **If you do not restore your key hormones to healthy, balanced levels, you will never cure your migraine.** That's how powerful the hormones are. I believe it's important for you to know all you can about each of the hormones associated with this debilitating condition and how you can harness their power to your advantage. That's what we are going to discuss in this chapter, with the help of several of the many patients who have learned how to be at home with their hormones.

It's amazing to me that although hormones have such a significant impact on health, our future physicians receive less than four hours of comprehensive training in medical school on the endocrine system and its various hormonal components. An exception are endocrinologists, physicians who elect to specialize in hormonal conditions and who are specially trained to diagnose and treat hormone problems in the body by restoring them to normal levels. Yet even these individuals are not attuned to the fact that hormonal imbalances can lead to chronic migraine headache. I am reminded of Arlene, who had been suffering with migraine for more than ten years before she started the program. She told me that she had visited an endocrinologist and asked him to check her estrogen, progesterone, testosterone, DHEA sulfate, and pregnenolone levels. The doctor dismissed her request, saying "I don't mess with those hormones." (One wonders exactly which hormones he does "mess with.")

Yet "those hormones" are critical when it comes to eliminating migraine. And so in this chapter I talk about the key hormones in the migraine story: what they are, the roles they play, and how to identify hormonal deficiencies and develop a hormone restoration program (with the help of a knowledgeable physician) that uses bio-identical supplements.

Hormones: Restoration, Replacement, Balance

Many people are familiar with the phrase "hormone replacement therapy," or HRT, especially as it relates to symptoms of perimenopause, menopause, and postmenopause or to its value as a preventive approach for bone density loss (osteoporosis) and possibly for macular degeneration, colon cancer, and delayed onset of Alzheimer's disease. Unfortunately, conventional HRT is also associated with an increased risk of heart attack, stroke, breast cancer, ovarian cancer, endometrial cancer, and gallbladder disease, among other conditions. We will talk about these risks later and how to avoid them.

First, however, I want to discuss the "star" of the Migraine Cure, *hormone restoration therapy*. The purpose of hormone restoration therapy is to restore certain hormones, which the body is unable to produce sufficient amounts of, to their **effective, optimal levels.** (You may recall our discussion in chapter 2 about optimal hormone levels and how important they are.) This approach is unlike hormone replacement, which replaces not only hormones the body can't produce, but also those it can. Hormone replacement can actually be detrimental, because it can cause the body to suppress its natural hormone production.

Testing for Hormone Levels

Before you can begin to balance your hormones, you will need to undergo a blood test to identify the levels of your basic steroid hormones. Once you have that information, you and your physician will have a reference point from which to begin restoration therapy. (A lipid [blood fats] panel is also done at this time to determine cholesterol levels.) For women who are still menstruating, who comprise the majority of migraineurs, the optimal time to take the test is during days 19 to 21 of the menstrual cycle, as this is the time progesterone levels peak. Test results obtained at this time will provide a clearer picture of the extent of hormone imbalance, especially with respect to estrogen and progesterone. Blood tests will need to be repeated a few more times, every few months or so depending on how well you follow the treatment plan and respond to it, to monitor hormone levels and help determine the optimal levels for you.

I know there are many health-care professionals who advocate saliva testing for determining hormone levels, and there are several facilities and numerous physicians who will conduct these tests for you. However, I recommend blood testing rather than saliva testing because the majority of people from their mid-thirties and older have some type of gum problems, even minor ones, that can secrete blood into saliva. Even a minute amount of blood in saliva can lead to inaccurate test results. Therefore, I strongly urge patients to choose blood testing for hormone levels.

Restoring Hormone Balance

While optimal hormone levels are critical, so is hormone balance. Thus the Migraine Cure strives to restore a balanced ratio between complementary hormones, such as estrogen and progesterone, and cortisol and DHEA, rather than restoring individual hormones to absolute numbers. As you'll see, achieving balanced ratios between certain hormones is critical for balancing the sympathetic and parasympathetic nervous systems which, as you'll recall, is an underlying goal of the Migraine Cure. When we restore—not replace—selected hormones and achieve a hormonal balance that is **specific to your unique body chemistry and needs**, then we can eliminate migraine.

I also want to reemphasize that elimination of migraine requires that we adjust the levels of all the hormones involved in migraine, not just one or two, as they have an intimate working relationship. Remember the car analogy: if you put air into just three of four tires, your car won't perform properly. Sometimes people start the migraine treatment program but decide they don't want to take one of the hormones or supplements because they want to "wait and see" what happens if they do just part of the treatment. What typically happens is that their migraines and associated symptoms improve—they may experience fewer or less intense migraines — but they don't go away. These patients limp along with one flat tire until they follow the complete plan.

There's another reason why we restore all five hormones instead of just a few: it allows us to use smaller doses of each one and ultimately gives us better control over the restoration and balancing process. We always want to use the lowest levels of hormones and other supplements possible that will allow us to reach out goals.

Now it's time to take a closer look at the genesis and life of the hormones involved in the Migraine Cure. First I talk about each of the hormones individually without giving dosing information. Then I bring the discussion of all five hormones together and talk about dosing, **because it is the balance among the hormones, and not their individual levels, that are critical to the elimination of migraine.** Thus any discussion of dosing should be done together.

Cholesterol: The First Ingredient

Before we look at the hormones, we need to examine cholesterol for a moment. In chapter 2, I showed you in a flow chart how the production of hormones begins with cholesterol. Therefore having a healthy level of cholesterol is critical for adequate hormone production. You may be thinking, "certainly having enough cholesterol in order to manufacture hormones shouldn't be a problem, because don't lots of people have *high* cholesterol?" And you are right; high cholesterol, or hypercholesterolemia, defined as 200 mg/dL or greater, affects about 107 million Americans, and about 20 percent of Americans have levels higher than 240 mg/dL.

The reason many people have high cholesterol is not because they are consuming a lot of high-cholesterol foods, but because the body responds to declining hormones levels (which occurs naturally as we age) by producing more and more cholesterol. But because the body does not use this cholesterol to manufacture more hormones, the blood levels of this artery-clogging substance increases instead. I and some of my colleagues believe that hypercholesterolemia, including so-called familial hypercholesterolemia, is the body's response to the decline or poor production of steroid hormones, and the solution is to balance the hormones, which in turn will lower cholesterol. Yet most physicians would rather prescribe cholesterol-lowering drugs, such as the statin drugs (e.g., atorvastatin [Lipitor®], simvastatin [Zocor®]), which, along with the fact that they can cause various side effects, can actually result in a hormone imbalance. (I talk more about the relationship between hormones and hypercholesterolemia in chapter 7.)

Abnormally low cholesterol is also a health problem. Research indicates that people who have levels of 160 mg/dL or lower have an increased risk of depression, anxiety, and suicide. Therefore, cholesterol levels that are too high or too low are unhealthy, including when it comes to balancing hormone levels. That's why when an individual with migraine wants to begin treatment, we always ask that he or she get a lipid panel (total cholesterol, LDL, HDL, and triglycerides) along with the hormone panel (discussed below).

Pregnenolone

If you did a random survey in a shopping mall or on the street and asked one hundred people what pregnenolone is, the most common response would likely be "preg what?" The fact is, pregnenolone is not only the most prevalent hormone in the brain, but it is also considered to be a "grandmother" hormone, one from which all the human steroid hormones, including aldosterone, cortisol, cortisone, DHEA, estrogen, progesterone, and testosterone are produced. (The term "steroid hormone" refers to a family of structurally similar biochemicals that have the ability to determine sex, reduce inflammation, and regulate growth.) Thus it follows that when levels of any of these hormones fall below normal, pregnenolone levels typically also are not normal, and vice versa.

Rare exceptions do occur, however. Of all the individuals who have participated in this migraine program, I have seen only two who have had normal pregnenolone levels. This is highly unusual in people who have migraine. One was Melissa, whom you met in chapter 1. Her case is a perfect example of how and why the Migraine Cure cannot be a one-size-fits-all program, and why it must be tailored for each individual and considers factors beyond the results of laboratory tests.

The Story of Pregnenolone

Pregnenolone is made from cholesterol. In a way, you could say that cholesterol is critical for your sex life: abnormally low levels of cholesterol translates into low production of pregnenolone, and thus low levels of sex hormones. The transformation of cholesterol to pregnenolone takes place mainly in the adrenal glands, but small amounts of pregnenolone are produced by the liver, skin, ovaries, testicles, brain, and retina of the eyes as well. This transformation or production process does not stay the same throughout your life. Production peaks in your early twenties, when the average adult makes about 14 mg per day, then declines gradually and steadily as the years pass. By age forty, you produce half the amount of the hormone that you made at twenty. Other factors that reduce the body's production of pregnenolone include stress, depression, exposure to environmental toxins, and hypothyroidism.

Scientists first began studying pregnenolone in the 1930s and looked at its effects on fatigue and autoimmune disorders, including rheumatoid arthritis, in the 1940s. Although pregnenolone proved to be safe and effective against rheumatoid arthritis, it is a natural substance and cannot be patented. Thus in 1949 when the pharmaceutical company Merck introduced cortisone to the general public to treat this disease, pregnenolone quickly faded into obscurity. Cortisone was soon followed by the synthetic steroid hormones dexamethasone and prednisone (and therefore both patentable and profit-producing), and these two agents were not only much more potent than pregnenolone, but faster acting and much more profitable. The advantages of the synthetic hormones were seriously challenged by their disadvantages, however. It seems that these unnatural hormones compromise the immune system as well as stimulate the development of osteoporosis. Although cortisone is a stress hormone produced by the body, the Merck product was given at amounts greater than is natural to the body, and so it was associated with risks similar to those linked to the synthetic steroid hormones.

I'm telling you this story about pregnenolone because it is a good example of how a natural, bio-friendly, beneficial agent **that cannot be patented**, is often sidelined to make room for patentable, profit-producing pharmaceuticals. The Migraine Cure involves use of natural, bio-friendly, nonpatentable agents *exclusively.*

Properties of Pregnenolone

As I mentioned previously, pregnenolone is one of the hormone levels that must be checked when an individual wishes to begin the Migraine Cure program. Few doctors check pregnenolone levels, however, and I believe this is a serious oversight. If you want to restore the levels of other hormones, such as estrogens, progesterone, and cortisol, you need to know a patient's pregnenolone level.

Here are some of the properties attributed to pregnenolone and some reasons why it is such an important hormone in the fight against migraine:

- Has the ability to normalize the levels of other hormones. Stress, for example, causes the release of excessive amounts of cortisol, a stress hormone. Cortisol is also known as the "death hormone" because chronically high levels are associated with accelerated aging and compromise of the immune system and can thus cause problems such as difficulties with memory, bone loss, fatigue, blood sugar irregularities, heart problems, and fat accumulation. Thus the decline in pregnenolone levels with age helps promote damage by cortisol, while supplementation of this steroid hormone regulates the negative impact of excess cortisol.
- Used by the brain to synthesize acetylcholine, a neurotransmitter that has a major role in the parasympathetic nervous system in transmitting nerve signals. Acetylcholine also plays a part in cognition, memory, and sleep.

- Helps with the formation of new brain cells, and thus has a positive impact on learning, concentration, and memory.
- Improves mood and relieves depressive symptoms. People who are depressed often have abnormally low levels of pregnenolone in their cerebrospinal fluid.
- Improves inflammation and allergies.
- Increases energy level. Fatigue is a common symptom of migraine.
- Relieves joint pain, spasticity, and tenderness associated with rheumatoid arthritis.
- Improves symptoms of premenstrual syndrome and menopause.

Taking Pregnenolone

Pregnenolone supplements are manufactured from wild yams *(Dioscorea villosa)* and are bio-identical to the hormone that your body produces naturally. Supplements are available in capsule form and as a sublingual tablet, and recommended doses are determined individually to meet each person's needs. Generally, however, the dosage is 50 to 200 mg daily, taken in the morning on an empty stomach, with the goal of attaining an optimal serum level (typical of a person age 20 to 29) of around 180 ng/dL for men or 200 ng/dL for women.

Pregnenolone is considered safe even at high doses. However, because pregnenolone is converted into DHEA and progesterone, which then are converted into other hormones, periodic blood testing of hormones is recommended, as we do in the Migraine Cure. This monitoring allows us to make any adjustments to your dose and to help ensure a healthy balance is reached among all the affected hormones.

DHEA

While pregnenolone is the grandmother of hormones—and the precursor of dehydroepiandrosterone (DHEA)—DHEA is the mother, because it is a precursor for the estrogens and testosterone (see figures 2 and 3 in chapter 2). DHEA also is referred to as a regulator, because it has the ability to help the body balance itself, especially the hormones your body needs.

DHEA has the distinction of being the most abundant steroid hormone in the human body, but that honor is short-lived. DHEA levels peak when you reach your early to mid twenties, then begin to decline steadily. By age 85, you can expect to have about only 5 percent of your optimal youthful level of DHEA. And with declining DHEA levels comes some negative health issues.

Most people are probably familiar with DHEA because since the early 1990s it has been widely touted in the media as an antiaging hormone. While low levels of DHEA are associated with aging, they also have been linked with various health problems, including but not limited to migraine, chronic inflammation, depression, rheumatoid arthritis, memory and concentration difficulties, osteoporosis, heart disease (in men), increased risk for some cancers, and complications of type 2 diabetes. On the positive side, taking DHEA supplements to restore the hormone to youthful levels can help treat many of these same conditions. That's why restoration of DHEA levels is part of the Migraine Cure.

The Power of DHEA

One of the main functions of DHEA is to counteract the stress-damaging actions of cortisol. Thus the ratio or balance of DHEA to cortisol is an important one to watch. The relationship between these two hormones becomes even more critical when you know that while DHEA levels decline with age, cortisol levels do not. In fact, cortisol levels can actually increase with age, especially in the presence of chronic or prolonged stress. That elevated level is often short-lived, however. My clinical experience shows that many migraine patients have lower than optimal cortisol levels because they are in adrenal fatigue (see chapter 2), due to the chronic stress that has exhausted their adrenal function. This became especially evident during an analysis I performed on 246 individuals who had various health conditions (e.g., fatigue, migraine, insomnia, depression, and so on) and who underwent a cortisol test. Only fourteen patients (5.7%) had slightly elevated cortisol levels.

Maintaining a high DHEA to optimal cortisol ratio is not only a critical key to anti-aging, but also important for achieving hormone balance and eliminating migraine. An imbalance between these two hormones also causes insulin levels to rise, which is a risk factor for diabetes and heart attack. Thus there are many good reasons to restore your DHEA levels and the DHEA-cortisol ratio, and the best way to do so is through supplementation.

Testing For and Taking DHEA

Your body's production of DHEA can be reliably identified by measuring the amount of DHEA sulfate (DHEA-S) in a blood sample. (DHEA-S is one of the levels measured when blood is taken as part of a basic steroid hormone panel.) The goal of DHEA supplementation is to restore levels to their youthful (age 20 to 29) range. For men the optimal range is 500 to 640 ug/dL; for women, 250 to 380 ug/dL. What is optimal for one person is not for another, so it is common for individuals to try several different doses to help them achieve their optimal range. The usual daily dose is 50 to 100 mg taken as an oral supplement, but as you'll see in the stories of patients throughout this book, adjustments of the DHEA dose are often necessary to meet an individual's needs.

Once the hormonal level has been restored, it is necessary to continue taking DHEA at this dose to maintain an optimal blood level. In people who are younger than thirty-five who have reached their optimal DHEA level through supplementation and who have remained migraine-free for three to four months, it is possible for them to discontinue DHEA for one month. After one month, they need to recheck their blood levels of DHEA, and if their body continues to maintain the optimal level, they can refrain from taking DHEA for as long as their level remains good. Naturally, this varies from person to person, and I strongly recommend that these younger individuals continue to monitor their DHEA levels regularly.

Because DHEA is a precursor for the estrogens and testosterone, it can have some effect on increasing the levels of these hormones. That's why it's important for women to undergo periodic blood tests to have the levels of these hormones checked.

There is some debate about the best way to take DHEA. Some experts say taking it with fat (e.g., avocado, peanut butter) helps the body assimilate the hormone better, while others say the supplement is better absorbed when taken on an empty stomach about 30 minutes before a meal. I recommend the second approach, with the meal being breakfast. If you need to take DHEA twice a day, which is usually a temporary measure, then the second dose should be taken before lunch.

There's no disagreement, however, about the best time of day to take DHEA: early in the day to prevent possible insomnia and other sleep disturbances. When you take DHEA early in the morning, you simulate your body's natural DHEA cycle: the adrenal glands produce the hormone early in the day and then it is converted by the liver to DHEA-S by midday when the DHEA-to-DHEA-S ratio usually reaches its balance of 10% DHEA and 90% DHEA-S.

Safety of DHEA

One question that frequently comes up when we recommend DHEA restoration to individuals is whether it is safe, as its use is sometimes associated with side effects. The answer is that DHEA is safe if we simultaneously restore the two basic female hormones—estrogen and progesterone—to optimal levels, and we block the undesirable conversion of testosterone to dihydrotestosterone (DHT). (For the blocked conversion, we use saw palmetto, which I discuss below.) In women, doses of DHEA greater than 50 to 100 mg per day may cause unwanted symptoms such as the development of facial hair, oily skin, or acne. If any of these symptoms occur, the dose of DHEA can be decreased, and the symptoms disappear.

Quite often we also recommend that individuals take 7-keto DHEA in addition to a regular DHEA supplement. 7-keto DHEA is a metabolite of

DHEA (a product of DHEA metabolism). Perhaps the most important feature of 7-keto is the fact that, unlike DHEA, it does not convert to estrogen and testosterone. Therefore, availability of the supplement 7-keto DHEA allows you to take a lower dose of DHEA (and thus reduce or eliminate the risk of developing side effects), which has the ability to help balance estrogen and progesterone levels and to keep cortisol levels in check.

It's important to remember that the hormone doses we recommend as part of the Migraine Cure, including those for DHEA, are often high at the beginning of treatment (especially when individuals are taking heavy doses of prescription drugs), but that we reduce them usually after two or four weeks as the body begins to regain balance. Several studies of DHEA in which 50 mg was given daily for one year showed the hormone supplement to be safe and having a "lack of harmful consequences."

Estrogen And Progesterone

Estrogen and progesterone are produced naturally by the body and typically thought of as female sex hormones. Indeed, females typically have higher levels of these two hormones than do males, but both estrogen and progesterone are found in people of both sexes and of all ages.

The roles of estrogen and progesterone in migraine are both critical and complex. I have grouped these two hormones together because they are so intimately connected, and because we have found that it is the **balance between them,** and not the restoration of optimal levels individually, that is critical for elimination of migraine, as well as the many symptoms women experience during perimenopause and menopause, as I discuss below.

To get an idea of the effects of estrogen and progesterone, see the accompanying table. You can see that these two hormones complement each other, with estrogen stimulating the sympathetic nervous system and progesterone promoting activity of the parasympathetic nervous system. Another way to say this is, estrogen excites the brain, while progesterone calms it. In addition, these two hormones are important separately to our discussion of migraine, and so I talk about their individual characteristics as well.

ESTROGEN AND PROGESTERONE BALANCING

Indications of Estrogen Dominance
- Occurrence of cyclical migraine
- Increase in body fat and weight
- Retention of fluids and salt; bloating
- Feelings of anxiety
- Depression
- Sleep difficulties
- Increased risk of blood clots

- Decline in sex drive
- Causes endometrial cancer

- Helps prevent bone loss

- Increased risk of prostate cancer
- Increased risk of breast cancer

- Loss of zinc and retention of copper

Effects of Progesterone
- Helps prevent migraine
- Helps burn fat
- Natural diuretic

- Has calming effect
- Natural antidepressant
- Aids normal sleep
- Helps normalize blood clotting
- Helps restore libido
- Helps prevent endometrial cancer

- Stimulates formation of new bone
- Helps reduce risk
- Helps prevent breast cancer

- Normalizes these levels

INDICATIONS OF PROGESTERONE DEFICIENCY OR IMBALANCE

- Menstrual difficulties
- Autoimmune disorders; e.g., lupus, rheumatoid arthritis, fibromyalgia
- Loss of bone density (premenopausal)
- Fibrocystic breasts

- Uterine cancer
- Ovarian cancer
- Osteoporosis (postmenopausal)

Estrogen Dominance

In the above table I introduce the term "estrogen dominance," which is very important to our discussion and is a term that is often misunderstood. Many people think estrogen dominance means the presence of an extremely high level of estrogen, but it can also mean a situation in which estrogen levels are normal and progesterone levels are low, or when estrogen levels are low and progesterone is very low. In all these situations, the result is an imbalance between these two critical hormones.

What causes estrogen dominance? Genetics can play a role, as some women have a natural tendency to produce higher levels of estrogen. However, other factors typically play a greater role and include:

- A decline in progesterone production, which can occur when a woman fails to ovulate (see discussion below).
- Excess (28% or greater) body fat. Fat cells produce estrogen; the more fat you have, the more estrogen your body produces.
- Excess stress, which results in elevated cortisol, insulin, and norepinephrine levels, which in turn lead to adrenal fatigue.
- Low-fiber diet and/or high intake of refined carbohydrates.
- Impaired liver function.
- Exposure to xenoestrogens, substances in the environment that act like estrogens in the body and can alter hormone levels. One of the most common ways you are exposed to xenoestrogens is through the pesticides used on commercially grown fruits and vegetables; another is through the hormones in meat and dairy products. Other sources include contaminated drinking water, leakage into food from plastics (especially plastic wraps on meats and dairy products and from plastic water bottles), through your skin from use of lotions, shampoos, cosmetics, and solvents; and from pesticides and herbicides used in your home, garden, and public places.

You can also see in the table that many of the indications of estrogen dominance are symptoms associated with migraine. When we take a closer look at, say, retention of fluids and salt, the scenario goes like this: estrogen dominance causes the body to retain sodium, which in turn leads to fluid retention and edema (bloating). Decreasing levels of progesterone is another reason for the development of edema, yet if we add progesterone as part of hormone restoration therapy, it has a diuretic action and balances estrogen. Another cause of fluid retention is low levels of luteinizing hormone, which, as you'll recall, is the hormone that is released from the pituitary and transported to the adrenals, where it stimulates production of progesterone. Thus again you can see the close relationship many of the components of the Migraine Cure have with each other and that it's important for all of them to function at their best in order to eliminate migraine.

Hormone Replacement Controversy

Over the past few years, there has been increasing controversy over the use, safety, and effectiveness of estrogen alone and hormone replacement therapy, which includes both estrogen and progesterone. The majority of the debates have centered around the use of these hormone therapies in women who are experiencing symptoms of perimenopause and menopause and the risk of coronary heart disease, stroke, and various cancers, and sprung up because of the results of the Women's Health Initiative (WHI). As I mentioned in chapter 3, the WHI's findings struck fear into women and many health-care professionals about the safety of estrogen and hormone replacement therapy.

Yet clear-thinking researchers and clinicians recognized that it was a combination of the unnatural use of unnatural hormones that fueled the negative findings of the study and the inaccurate message that estrogen was "bad." Fortunately, more and more studies are coming out in support of the use of bio-identical hormones given to simulate natural hormone cycles for menopause and now, migraine, although the positive message is slow to catch on. And as you've already learned, bio-identical estrogen and progesterone are crucial elements in the development and elimination of migraine. Let's take a closer look at these two hormones.

A Trio of Power: The Estrogens

"Estrogen" is actually a blanket term for several types of the hormone, of which three — estriol, estradiol, and estrone — are the most important. Production of estrogens involves the cooperation of several elements. It begins with the hypothalamus (remember the HPA axis discussed in chapter 2), which releases gonadotropin-releasing hormone (GnRH), which travels to the pituitary gland, where it stimulates the release of follicle-stimulating hormone (FSH), which causes the release of a follicle, which in turn prompts the secretion of estrogens.

Estrogens perform a great many functions in the body, a fact evidenced by the presence of more than three hundred different types of estrogen receptors in the female body, all of which can be activated by estrogen. This means many different functions in a woman's body respond to estrogen and its fluctuating levels, which explains, for example, the numerous and diverse symptoms that are associated with premenstrual syndrome.

When the three estrogens are present in the proper balance with each other and with other steroid hormones, health and well-being are maintained. Indications of an estrogen deficiency are all-too familiar to women who are entering menopause: night sweats, sleep problems, poor memory, irritability, vaginal dryness, and hot flashes, among other symptoms. Women are also aware that an estrogen deficiency is associated with a high risk of osteoporosis, and increasing evidence is pointing toward a link with the development of Alzheimer's disease.

At the other end of the spectrum are signs of estrogen dominance, which are the same factors associated with the use of estrogen therapy and HRT: an increased risk of breast cancer, endometrial cancer, blood clots, heart disease, stroke, and gallbladder disease. In fact, estrogen dominance stimulates the sympathetic nervous system, which, as you'll recall, is responsible for raising blood pressure and heart rate and other stress-related, "fight or flight" reactions in the body (see chapter 1). Estrogen dominance is also associated with migraine.

All three estrogens work together to support the central nervous system, determine female physical characteristics, minimize loss of calcium from bone, enhance skin health, promote blood clotting, and support ovulation, among other functions. Yet although all three play critical roles in the body, they are not equal in terms of safety or benefits.

Estradiol and estrone, for example, along with their positive features, have cancer-causing abilities, and the body naturally allows for this negative characteristic by producing lower levels of these estrogens compared with the so-called "good" estrogen, estriol. In fact, estriol is believed to have cancer-reducing properties. Thus, the normal, healthy breakdown of total estrogens in women is 60 to 80 percent estriol, and 10 to 20 percent each of estradiol and estrone. Keep these percentages in mind, as they are the guidelines we use when recommending natural estrogens to women who participate in the Migraine Cure.

Estrogen levels are in a state of constant flux, especially in women during their reproductive years. This span of time, from adolescence to menopause around the mid-century mark, is also when women are most likely to have migraine. Estrogen levels in normal, healthy women basically follow this pattern during a 28-day menstrual cycle: estrogen levels are

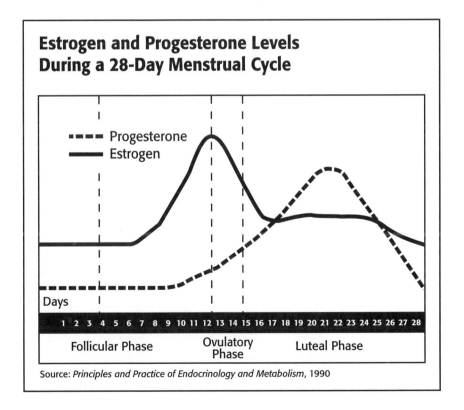

Estrogen and Progesterone Levels During a 28-Day Menstrual Cycle

- - - - Progesterone
——— Estrogen

Days

1 2 3 4 5 6 7 8 9 10 11 12 13 14 15 16 17 18 19 20 21 22 23 24 25 26 27 28

Follicular Phase | Ovulatory Phase | Luteal Phase

Source: *Principles and Practice of Endocrinology and Metabolism*, 1990

lowest during menstruation, after which they rise rapidly near midcycle and fall just before ovulation (around days 12 through 15 of the cycle). During the next two weeks (days 16 through 28), estrogen levels remain low while progesterone, which is produced only after ovulation and peaks at around day 22, is dominant. Progesterone then declines rapidly before menstruation. Overall, estrogen dominates during the first two weeks of the cycle, with low levels of progesterone acting as a balance; and progesterone dominates during the second two weeks, with low estrogen balancing.

ESTROGEN AND MIGRAINE

The relationship between estrogen levels and the development and elimination of migraine is an intimate one. Here is what we know about estrogen and migraine:

- The prevalence of migraine increases at menarche (when a female's menstrual cycle first begins).
- The decline in estrogen levels just before menstruation triggers migraine in many women.
- Migraines usually decline during the second and third trimesters of pregnancy when estrogen levels are high.
- Migraines commonly occur immediately after a women gives birth as estrogen levels decline dramatically.
- Migraines generally improve or disappear with natural (but not surgically induced) menopause, which is characterized by a decline in **both** estrogen and progesterone (more on progesterone below).
- Fluctuations of estrogen levels result in changes in melatonin secretion and in neurotransmitters such as serotonin, noradrenaline, and endorphins, the body's natural pain killers. All of these elements have a role in migraine.

TAKING ESTROGEN

The form of bio-identical estrogen that I recommend is Triest® gel, which I recommend be taken in a formulation that consists of 90 percent estriol, 7 percent estradiol, and 3 percent estrone. A compounding pharmacy can prepare this specific formulation for you. This formulation is most advantageous for women, especially those older than thirty-five, because it provides a large percentage of safe estrogen—estriol—which I discuss below, along with the other two types of estrogen.

- Estriol: This is a weak estrogen, therefore larger amounts must be given as restoration therapy. It is also the safer estrogen, because it is not associated with the increased risk of breast and ovarian cancer attributed to estradiol and estrone. In fact, pioneering research by Dr. HM Lemon of the University of Nebraska Medical Center found that estriol can help prevent breast cancer.

- Estrone: Estrone sulphate is the form of estrogen used in the prescription hormone drug Premarin, which is made from the urine of pregnant mares. According to the *Merck Manual*, estrone is a known carcinogen, and it's been shown to cause a significantly increased risk of breast and ovarian cancer if it is used for more than 10 years.

- Estradiol: Like estrone, estradiol has been identified as a known carcinogen when it is present in unbalanced, inappropriate amounts. The form of the hormone found in the prescription drugs Estrace and Estraderm is 17-beta estradiol.

This gel should be applied in the morning after bathing, to areas such as the vulva (best absorption is achieved at this site), neck, forearm, or sides of the chest or abdomen. Although you may have read or heard that you should change the application site each day, there is no need to do so.

Nancy's Story

Estrogen dominance and a significant estrogen/progesterone imbalance is very common among people who have migraine, and Nancy was no exception. When Nancy first sought help from us in 1999, she was forty-eight years old and had been experiencing eight or nine migraines per month for more than ten years. She also suffered from high cholesterol, high blood pressure, depression, sleeping problems, irritability, fatigue, low sex drive, poor short-term memory, genital herpes, arthritis, and irregular menstrual periods, the latter which was associated with perimenopause. She has two sons, both of whom were away at college, and she worked part-time as a medical records clerk in a dentist's office near her home in downtown Chicago, a job that allowed her some flexibility when migraines made it impossible for her to go to the office.

At 5'5" and 130 pounds, Nancy was at a healthy weight, and although she said she wanted to lose a few pounds, she also confessed to being too tired most of the time to exercise. At the time, she was taking several prescription medications for high blood pressure (Procardia XL and Nifedical XL), hot flashes (Premphase, which contains synthetic estrogen and synthetic progestin), insomnia (zolpidem, Ambien®), depression (sertraline, Zoloft®), and genital herpes (Zovirax and Valtrex), but no prescription drugs for migraine, which she said she treated with "high doses of several over-the-counter products."

> Her initial lipid and hormone profiles revealed the following levels. (Reference ranges are in parentheses.)
> - Total estrogen: 643 pg/mL (61-437 pg/mL) (Note that in females, total estrogen levels are measured; in males, only estradiol is measured.)
> - Total testosterone: 29 ng/dL (14-76 ng/dL)
> - Progesterone: 0.7 (0.2-28 ng/mL)
> - DHEA-S: 66 ug/dL (65-380 ug/dL)
> - Pregnenolone: 50 (10-230 ng/dL)
> - Total cholesterol: 241 mg/dL (<200 mg/dL)

Nancy had a significant hormone imbalance, with very high total estrogen and very low progesterone, leaving her with a highly unbalanced ratio between these two hormones (estrogen dominance), as well as low pregnenolone and DHEA-S levels. These are common findings among people with migraine. Her estrogen dominance, which can stimulate the sympathetic nervous system and thus cause an imbalance with the parasympathetic system, was likely the reason why her blood pressure was not under control (150/90 mmHg) even though she was taking two blood pressure medications. Her cholesterol level also was high, again a common finding in people whose hormones are out of balance (see chapter 8). We immediately suggested the following plan for hormone restoration. All hormones were taken in the morning:

- Estrogen: a gel (Triest®) compounded to contain 90% estriol, 7% estradiol, and 3% estrone. The recommended dose was 0.6 mL on days 1 through 10 following her menstrual period, then 0.4 mL on days 11 through 21.
- Progesterone: micronized gel (50 mg/mL) at a dose of 0.6 mL on days 1 through 10 following her menstrual period, then 0.8 mL
- Testosterone: micronized gel (50 mg/mL) at a dose of 0.1 mL daily.
- Pregnenolone: 100 mg daily in the morning.
- DHEA: 50 mg daily in the morning.

Along with the hormones, we recommended Nancy take the following supplements:

- A proprietary high-potency vitamin/mineral/bioflavonoid/herbal mix, 3 tablets three times daily.
- Omega-3 fatty acids, 1,000 mg in the morning
- A probiotic combination product that contains 3.5 billion *Lactobacillus* group (*L. rhamnosus A, L. rhamnosus B, L. acidophilus, L. casei, L. bulgaricus*), 1.0 billion *Bifidobacterium* group (*B. longum, B. breve*), and 0.5 billion *Streptococcus* ther-

mophilus, as well as gluten-free grasses, algae, natural fiber, herbs, and bioflavonoid extracts: one scoop in the morning.

- Glucosamine sulfate, 2,000 mg in the morning. Glucosamine is a substance produced by the body (and also available as a supplement) that rehabilitates cartilage and is helpful in treating the pain of arthritis.
- Phosphatidylserine, 200 mg in the morning (this was for short-term memory improvement).

Nancy was very enthusiastic about the program and was anxious to begin. After her third day of treatment, she told her primary care physician that she was stopping Premphase, but she continued to take her other medications. By the end of the fourth week of treatment, Nancy reported that she had had only two migraines instead of her usually eight or nine, and that they both had been much less severe than normal. Her blood pressure had dropped to 130/90 mmHg, and her arthritis pain was completely gone.

Although her migraines had improved, it was obvious we needed to make some adjustments to her hormone restoration therapy to reach our goal. We recommended that she change her DHEA dose to 100 mg in the morning and 50 mg at noon, taken an additional 0.2 mL of progesterone before going to bed, and add 420 mg of magnesium citrate to be taken one hour before bedtime. She said she would make the changes and let us know the outcome.

Nancy contacted us again in three months and was beside herself. Her migraines were gone, and so was her depression and anxiety, so she had stopped taking Zoloft and Ambien. Her blood pressure had continued to improve, so her primary care physician had discontinued one of her blood pressure medications. Nancy said she felt so good and had so much energy, she had begun to exercise about four times a week. At this point we recommended she reduce her DHEA to 50 mg taken in the morning and increase her pregnenolone to 200 mg in the morning.

One year after she started treatment, Nancy says she feels like a new person. "My family and friends can't believe the difference in me," she said.

"I feel like I've restarted living life. I'm migraine-free and I don't need any of the medications I was taking before." Nancy continues to take hormone restorative therapy and several supplements. She enjoys a healthy cholesterol level (187 mg/dL), a safe blood pressure for which she no longer needs medication (120-130/70 mmHg), and has had no recurrence of depression, arthritis symptoms, or herpes.

Progesterone: The "Other" Female Hormone

As you have probably noticed, it's hard to talk about estrogen and its role in migraine without also talking about progesterone. The balance between estrogen and progesterone is critical in the elimination of migraine, and so let's look a little closer at how this important hormone works.

Progesterone levels in the body naturally rise and fall during a woman's monthly cycle. Production of progesterone, which occurs in the ovaries of women who ovulate (release of a ripe egg from the ovary), begins just before ovulation, increases rapidly after ovulation, and remains at a high level, about 20 to 25 mg daily, for the last two weeks of the menstrual cycle. Women who do not ovulate do not produce progesterone in their ovaries—either because their ovaries have been removed, they have amenorrhea (lack of menstruation), or they are postmenopausal — although small amounts are always being made by the adrenal glands and fat cells.

Women can begin to miss ovulations as early as their mid thirties, and missed ovulations become more common as perimenopause approaches. (Note that during perimenopause [ages 30-50] women can get their period even if they do not ovulate. Thus a woman may think she is still producing progesterone when in fact she is not.) The combination of missed ovulations and the approach of menopause usually results in progressively lower levels of progesterone, which contributes to an imbalance with estrogen, whose levels are also always changing. This imbalance explains why many women begin to experience symptoms of perimenopause in their mid to late thirties and forties, and also why the peak incidence of migraine for women is between the ages of 35 and 45.

The fact that progesterone plays a role in eliminating migraine is not news. In 1953, Drs. Katharina Dalton and Raymond Greene reported that progesterone injections relieved migraines associated with women's menstrual cycle, as well as other symptoms of premenstrual syndrome (PMS). Decades later, Dr. Joel Hargrove at Vanderbilt University reported a 90 percent success rate in relieving symptoms of PMS when he treated women with a daily dose of oral micronized estradiol and progesterone.

Another interesting observation is the relationship between progesterone, estrogen, and magnesium. Magnesium has the ability to relax vascular smooth muscles, thus it is often recommended to relieve premenstrual symptoms, including headache, and it in fact plays a major role in the Migraine Cure. Although we discuss magnesium's role in migraine in depth later in chapter 7, here it's worth noting that migraine, especially in women, is associated with a deficiency of ionized magnesium. Research shows that as estrogen levels rise, ionized magnesium decreases, yet when progesterone levels rise, ionized magnesium levels also increase, a good argument for keeping these two substances at healthy, balanced levels in the body.

One more item of note about progesterone is its relationship to nitric oxide. Briefly, nitric oxide can be both beneficial and damaging to the body. For migraineurs who are supersensitive to nitric oxide, the relationship between progesterone and nitric oxide is positive, and I talk more about that relationship in chapter 5.

Types of Progesterone

When we talk about progesterone therapy or supplementation, there are two types available: bio-identical progesterone, which is chemically the same as the progesterone produced by the human body and thus behaves like the body's natural progesterone; and synthetic progesterone-like substances called progestogens or progestins. We looked at progestins in chapter 3 where I talked about hormone replacement therapy. The majority of clinical trials have used progestins (usually as medroxyprogesterone acetate [Provera®, Cycrin®]), which is also the type most physicians prescribe to women for symptoms of PMS and menopause, and in birth control pills. Now we look at the type of progesterone used in the Migraine Cure, bio-identical progesterone.

In the 1930s, a chemistry professor from Pennsylvania named Russell Marker was experimenting with plant steroids in Mexico when he discovered a process for producing natural progesterone. Marker found that natural progesterone supplements could be produced from a plant steroid called diosgenin (diosgenin is a so-called phytoestrogen; "phyto" means plant) which is found in the wild Mexican yam and soybeans. All that was needed was a simple molecular adjustment, which then made it identical to the progesterone produced naturally by the body.

One of the first people to discover the benefits of natural progesterone was Dr. John Lee, who, back in the 1970s, saw many menopausal women in his practice who could not take estrogen because of the significant risk of serious conditions such as heart disease, cancer, and diabetes. He became interested in research indicating that progesterone, not estrogen, would be most helpful to these women. When he recommended natural progesterone cream to his patients for symptoms of menopause, they reported relief from hot flashes, insomnia, bladder problems, dry eyes, irritability, hair loss, sore breasts, night sweats, and bloating, among other symptoms. After a few years, Dr. Lee realized that these women were also experiencing improved bone density as a result of taking progesterone.

Contrast these benefits of natural progesterone with the effects of progestins, which are chemically different from natural progesterone. In addition to not functioning effectively as natural progesterone in the body, they can also cause side effects. Although each synthetic progestin can cause different side effects, some of them include suppression of so-called good cholesterol (HDL), increased tendency to develop male characteristics (e.g., appearance of facial hair, deepening voice), elevation of blood pressure, and depression.

Taking Progesterone

The formulation of natural progesterone I recommend and use in the Migraine Cure is micronized progesterone USP. Micronization of progesterone is a process that produces minute crystals of progesterone, which are more readily and steadily absorbed from the gastrointestinal tract or through the skin. In the United States, the Upjohn Company provides micronized progesterone as a bulk powder to compounding pharmacies, where pharmacists specially prepare tablets or capsules for consumers in doses that have been specifically prescribed for them by their physicians to meet their particular needs. Micronized progesterone is also available as a gel (transdermal form), which is the form I recommend for migraine as well as other conditions that benefit from hormone balancing.

If the transdermal form is not available to you, oral natural progesterone is available. The Food and Drug Administration (FDA) approved Prometrium®, an oral pill that contains 100 and 200 mg of natural progesterone. But because oral progesterone is metabolized by the liver, people who have liver conditions should talk to their doctor before using this form of the hormone. Another problem with oral natural progesterone is that only 10 to 15 percent of the oral form reaches the bloodstream, thus you need to take five to seven times the dose of transdermal natural progesterone to get the same benefits. Yet one more problem with the oral form is that you cannot titrate (adjust) the dose up or down as your body requires.

The acronym USP stands for United States Pharmacopoeia, a national standard of purity for substances that are used in the production of cosmetics and drugs. Micronized progesterone that has USP on the label is your guarantee that the progesterone in the product has been converted to be bio-identical to the progesterone produced by the human body. Gels that contain wild yam extract (diogenin) only but no USP progesterone are not effective because the body cannot convert yam extracts into progesterone.

The base of progesterone gel should be an oil/water emulsion that also contains permeation enhancers, which increase the ability of the hormone to be transported beyond the skin barrier. The gel should be massaged into the vulva (an excellent absorption site) or into the soft tissue of the forearm or neck. The progesterone passes through the skin tissue, diffuses into the capillaries, and then reaches the general bloodstream. The micronized gel I recommend is available through compounding pharmacies, delivers 50 mg/mL, and should be applied in doses that simulate a woman's monthly cycle, as I explain in the stories I share with you in this book. In younger individuals (younger than thirty-five) an acceptable alternative is an over-the-counter cream product called ProFem, but I strongly recommend the micronized progesterone gel as the first choice when it is available.

HOW TO USE NATURAL PROGESTERONE

If you are woman using natural progesterone cream, it is critical that you apply it in a cycle that mimics a healthy woman's normal menstrual cycle. (Note: dosages given here are typical; however you may need different amounts based on your height, weight, deficiency symptoms, current levels, and any other specific requirements.) The cream should be applied in the morning to mimic the body's natural cycle. Because progesterone stimulates the parasympathetic nervous system (which dominates at night), some women and men find that applying about 25 percent of their daily dose at night is more in tune with their body's rhythms. These instructions apply to the over-the-counter product.

- If you are premenopausal, apply 1/3 teaspoon from the first day through the tenth day after menses have stopped; then use 1/2 teaspoon until the first day of menses.
- If you are postmenopausal, use 1/2 teaspoon for days 1 through 14, 3/4 teaspoon for days 15 through 25, and then 1/3 teaspoon for day 26 until the end of the month.

Testosterone

Testosterone is typically characterized as the male hormone, the one responsible for the normal development of male sex and reproductive organs, and development of secondary male sex traits, including hair growth (and loss) patterns, thickening of the vocal chord, muscle development, and other characteristics. Normal testosterone levels are necessary to maintain a healthy mood, energy level, bone marrow production, fertility, and sexual desire. Females also need testosterone; their levels need not be as high as those of males (see table in chapter 2), but their optimal levels should be sufficient to maintain good health. Testosterone levels need to be in balance to eliminate migraine in men and women as well.

In males, most of the testosterone is produced by the Leydig cells of the testes, which are stimulated into production by lutenizing hormone, secreted by the pituitary gland (see figure in chapter 1). A small amount is also made by steroids that are secreted by the adrenal cortex. Normal production of the testes is 4 to 7 milligrams of the hormone daily. Females, in contrast, make testosterone in their ovaries. In males, testosterone production increases rapidly at the beginning of puberty and decreases rapidly after age 50. Signs and symptoms of low testosterone levels in men include erectile dysfunction, low sex drive, depression, irritability, increased breast size, and weight gain (accumulation of abdominal fat).

Testing For and Using Testosterone

Measurement of testosterone levels is part of the male and female hormone panel that is used to identify the levels of other steroid hormones. Testosterone levels fluctuate from hour to hour, but the highest levels occur in the early morning. The optimal range for males is 650 to 827 ng/dL; for females, 60 to 76 ng/dL.

Testosterone supplements are available in oral form (capsules, pills), by injection, through a transdermal patch, and in a gel. I recommend the latter form because it allows for individualized dosing and is easy to use. In fact, the type of gel that we recommend is a PLO—a pluronic lecithin organo gel—which dries quickly and allows the testosterone to be readily absorbed into the skin, which then acts as a reservoir for the sustained release of the hormone into the bloodstream.

Patients sometimes want to use other forms of testosterone, which can be problematic and not provide the benefits of a gel. Oral forms, for example, are quickly absorbed into the bloodstream and then broken down by the liver, which means adequate levels of testosterone are not reached unless very high doses (40-50 mg/day) are taken. Unfortunately, high doses can cause liver damage and abnormal changes in blood lipids. Transdermal patches can cause itching, redness, or other irritation in some individuals, and they may also fall off when a person sweats. Injections need to be taken every seven to twenty-one days and cause a peak in testosterone blood levels two to three days after the injection, after which the levels slowly decline during the next one to two weeks. These fluctuations may be accompanied by mood changes.

Although it is necessary to balance testosterone levels with the other steroid hormones as part of the Migraine Cure, that balance is frequently achievable without an individual having to use a testosterone supplement (mostly in younger people). In women, correct levels of DHEA can convert into testosterone whenever the body recognizes that levels are low. Thus careful use of DHEA (a precursor of testosterone) restoration can help some women reach their optimal levels, while others do need a testosterone supplement, at least temporarily. Males, however, do not experience the same level of conversion of DHEA to testosterone. One migraineur who found that testosterone was especially important was Jonathan.

Jonathan's Story

Before he began experiencing migraines at age 23, Jonathan, who has his own management consulting company in a Milwaukee suburb, had always enjoyed good health. Yet for nearly fifteen years, he had been living with migraines, two to three per week, when he first contacted us. During those years he had also suffered with depression, fatigue, high cholesterol, and memory problems. He is fortunate in that he works for himself, so he could arrange his work schedule to end or to be interrupted in early to mid afternoon, as this was the time he typically experienced a migraine attack.

In the earlier years he had tried taking high doses of over-the-counter medications to deal with the migraines, then he tried several prescription drugs before finding that sumatriptan injections worked best for him. For the past eight years, he had been fairly successful in aborting attacks by taking these injections and then lying down for about fifteen minutes, but he was concerned about the number of injections (as many as six or seven) he needed in any given week to ward off the pain. Several years after starting the sumatriptan Jonathan began to take an antidepressant (Paxil, 20 mg daily) to ease his depression, fatigue, and poor memory. Despite the fact that he "can't be sure it really helps," he continued to take it until he started our program.

Both of Jonathan's parents have a long and continuous history of headache. His father suffers with chronic daily headache that he says are not migraine, but his mother experiences several migraines per year. Jonathan's medical history includes a vasectomy at age 29, which he says did not affect the frequency or severity of his migraines; and a diagnosis of high cholesterol at age 30, which prompted him to switch to a plant-based diet. Increasing lower back pain at age 34 caused him to undergo magnetic resonance imaging, which revealed a herniated disc and, of great concern to Jonathan, cartilage deterioration in all the discs in his back. This is a potential side effect associated with the use of sumatriptan, although Jonathan's neurologist did not believe there was a clear connection between use of the drug and the loss of cartilage. Jonathan was advised to continue taking sumatriptan, which he did reluctantly because, as he explained, "it allows me to work and have a somewhat normal life." He subsequently had surgery for the herniated disc and his back pain was significantly reduced, although he continued to worry that the sumatriptan was "eroding away my cartilage." His only consolation, he said, was that he found that he could take half the recommended dose of sumatriptan and usually still get enough relief to function.

Jonathan had been persistent in his search for better ways to treat his migraines. Over the years he went to at least half a dozen doctors and tried various supplements, including feverfew, magnesium, and butterbur extract, as well as an anticonvulsant that one doctor recommended. On several occasions he kept detailed notes on possible triggers, but he grew discouraged. "It seemed that everything was a trigger, from too much sleep to not enough sleep, wine, cheese, bright lights, using my computer, stress, weather changes, and on and on," he said. "There didn't seem to be a pattern."

Jonathan seemed more than ready to beat migraine when he first sought our help. After we spoke at length with him, we suggested he undergo blood testing, including a lipid profile. His results were as follows, with recommended ranges in parentheses:
- Cholesterol: 257 mg/dL (<200 mg/dL)
- Total testosterone: 187 ng/dL (241-827 ng/dL)

- Estradiol: 18 pg/dL (0-53 pg/dL) (Note that in males, estradiol levels alone, and not total estrogen levels, are measured)
- Progesterone: 1.6 ng/mL (0.3-1.2 ng/mL)
- Pregnenolone: <10 ng/dL (10-200 ng/dL)
- DHEA-S: 199 ug/dL (280-640 ug/dL)

Based on these results, we recommended the following:
- 100 mg pregnenolone taken in the morning
- 25 mg of DHEA taken in the morning
- 420 mg magnesium citrate taken at bedtime
- Melatonin formula for pineal gland balancing that contains 3 mg melatonin, 250 mg kava root extract, and 10 mg vitamin B6, taken at bedtime
- A probiotic combination product that contains 3.5 billion *Lactobacillus* group (*L. rhamnosus A, L. rhamnosus B, L. acidophilus, L. casei, L. bulgaricus*), 1.0 billion *Bifidobacterium* group (*B. longum, B. breve*), and 0.5 billion *Streptococcus thermophilus*, as well as gluten-free grasses, algae, natural fiber, herbs, and bioflavonoid extracts: one scoop in the morning
- Testosterone: We recommended a testosterone gel, as this hormone is necessary to restore a proper hormonal balance, but Jonathan declined, saying he wanted to wait a few weeks to see how he felt without the testosterone.

One week after Jonathan started treatment, he developed a fever of 102.7 degrees F and experienced night sweats. His primary care physician prescribed an antibiotic, and his symptoms disappeared in about a week. Jonathan was still getting migraines, and again we recommended that he consider testosterone restoration. He agreed to visit a urologist, who conducted an examination and said Jonathan's low testosterone levels could be the result of the vasectomy he had had years ago. At this point, five weeks after starting treatment, Jonathan agreed to give testosterone a try, and his urologist prescribed a 1% gel, which Jonathan applied daily. Within a week he was migraine-free and has remained so. He also reports that he has much more energy, his depression is gone, and that his sexual performance is much improved.

Jonathan's story illustrates the importance of restoring all the hormones to achieve balance and thus eliminate migraine. As long as Jonathan refused to add testosterone to the program, he was riding on only three inflated tires instead of four, to use the metaphor introduced earlier.

Treatment Enhancements: Zinc and Saw Palmetto

In males, saw palmetto (*Serenoa repens*), an herb that grows naturally in the southeastern United States, especially in Florida, Georgia, and Mississippi, is often used to help prevent prostate enlargement. That's because this herb blocks the conversion of testosterone to dihydrotestosterone (DHT), a substance which, among other things, stimulates growth of the prostate gland and causes hair loss. Specifically, saw palmetto inhibits the activity of 5-alpha-reductase, the enzyme that converts testosterone to DHT.

Use of saw palmetto to prevent prostate enlargement seems a far cry from recommending it for women who have migraine, but in fact it has proved quite useful for that purpose in selected cases. I discovered the connection in an interesting way.

Francine is a twenty-eight-year-old office manager who was extremely upset in 2002 when, over the course of a year, she gained nearly 200 pounds and lost nearly all of her thick, shoulder-length hair. She also was experiencing migraine, various premenstrual syndrome symptoms (e.g., irritability, mood swings, bloating), and an irregular menstrual cycle. Both hair loss and weight gain are two indications of testosterone dominance, and so I was not surprised when Francine's hormone profile results showed very high testosterone and DHT. She also had a deficiency of DHEA, progesterone, and pregnenolone.

Because Francine had symptoms caused by elevated DHT levels, I knew it would be necessary to block the conversion of testosterone to its metabolite, but how? Although the steroid hormone balance differs between males and females, the biochemistry is similar. Therefore, even though saw palmetto is typically used in males to block this conversion, I believed it would do the same thing in females. So we recommended that Francine take pregnenolone, DHEA, progesterone, saw palmetto, and zinc. The zinc was recommended because it can block aromatase enzyme, the factor that converts testosterone into estrogen. The addition of zinc could help prevent estrogen dominance and also facilitate an estrogen/progesterone balance.

Francine was highly motivated to begin the program, and her enthusiasm paid off almost immediately. Within a few weeks her migraines were gone, her PMS symptoms were nearly resolved, and her hair started to grow back. One year after she started hormone restoration, her hair was thick and full once again and she had lost 100 pounds. To this day she has remained migraine-free, her menstrual cycle is normal, and she continues to slowly lose weight toward her goal.

Most individuals who participate in the Migraine Cure need to take saw palmetto and/or zinc. When a female has symptoms that are associated with testosterone dominance, supplementing with this herb and nutrient can be beneficial. The typical dose of saw palmetto is 160 mg once daily, while the dose of zinc can range from 15 to 90 mg.

In Conclusion

Hormone restoration is the bedrock of the Migraine Cure. To get results, you *must* restore hormonal balance and you must use bio-identical hormones to achieve it. Doing anything less will leave you limping along on three tires. That's why if you don't understand something in this chapter, if you have questions, if you're still not convinced, please read on! (Actually, please read on anyway; there's much more to talk about the Migraine Cure.) In the next few chapters I explain how the other components of the Migraine Cure synchronize with the hormonal segment, and I share a few more stories about former migraineurs who have found relief at last—and how you can, too.

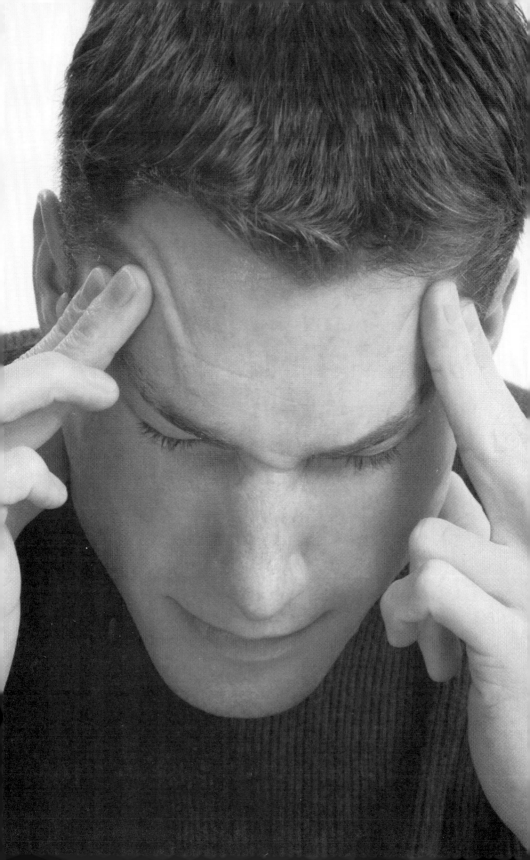

5

Resetting The Pineal Gland

It may be only the size of a pea, but the pineal gland, located deep in the brain, plays a major role in both the development and elimination of migraine. That's because this tiny gland is the body's primary source of melatonin, a hormone that orchestrates the body's circadian (daily) rhythm, including and especially sleep patterns. What does migraine have to do with melatonin and circadian rhythm? Plenty. As far back as the mid 1980s, researchers had made some clinical observations and posed the following question: "Is migraine due to a deficiency of pineal melatonin?" Indeed, today we know that migraine is a response to irregularities in the pineal circadian cycle. This piece of information, along with the fact that various sleep disturbances trigger migraine in many migraineurs, have been instrumental in my belief that it is necessary to normalize or balance the pineal circadian cycle in order to eliminate migraine and its related symptoms, including sleep disorders.

In this chapter, I explain how you can achieve these goals. To do that, we will look at the body's circadian rhythm cycle and the roles that the pineal gland, serotonin, melatonin, and several other factors play in the development and elimination of migraine and migraine-related symptoms, and the relationship between the activities of the pineal gland and the other components of the Migraine Cure.

Insomnia: More Than Feeling Tired

Insomnia is no stranger to people who have migraine. In fact, the vast majority of migraineurs experience insomnia or some sort of sleep disturbance regularly. Insomnia is a sleep disorder characterized by difficulty falling asleep or staying asleep, or failing to feel rested after a night's sleep (or trying to sleep). Besides the fatigue and mental fogginess that accompany a lack of sufficient sleep, sleep deprivation or sleeping at odd hours, as in people who work nights, has been linked with an increased risk of serious health problems, including heart disease, obesity, diabetes, hypertension, and cancer. It's also been associated with an increased prevalence of emotional and psychological problems, a higher mortality rate, and more frequent hospitalizations.

Clearly, insomnia is about more than being tired. One possible explanation for these associated health problems is that they are consequences of the chronic stress and overstimulation of the sympathetic nervous system that go hand-in-hand with insufficient sleep. For example, studies show that sleep deprivation in healthy individuals causes an imbalance between the sympathetic and parasympathetic nervous systems; in fact, it results in activation of the sympathetic nervous system, which is counterproductive to sleep. Insufficient sleep results in a disruption in the secretion of cortisol (the stress hormone) and in endocrine function, which is critical for migraine because the endocrine glands (e.g., pituitary, pineal, adrenal) are key producers of hormones involved in migraine. Lack of sleep also can cause an increase in blood pressure, and fluctuations in lipid and glucose metabolism. The imbalance in the sympathetic and parasympathetic nervous systems and disruption in endocrine function are of especial interest to us, as they are characteristic of migraine. Therefore, you can see that insomnia and related sleep disturbances are an important factor in our discussion of migraine.

Migraine And Sleep

"I'm never sure exactly what's going to trigger an attack," says Gwen, a forty-eight-year-old real estate broker. "Sometimes too little sleep triggers a migraine and sometimes too much sleep sets one off. Whenever I don't get enough sleep I worry that I'm going to get a migraine. Yet I'm tired so much of the time, that when I try to sleep in, I worry that too much sleep will give me a migraine as well. Sleep is a real problem for me."

Sleep as a Trigger

Gwen's problems with sleep and their relationship to her migraines are far from unusual. According to the results of a study of more than 1,700 migraine patients conducted by Leslie Kelman, MD, medical director at the Headache Center of Atlanta, and presented at the American Headache Society's 47th Annual Scientific Meeting, 75 percent of migraineurs report they have triggers that set off an acute migraine attack. Of these individuals, 50 percent of them list sleep disturbances as a trigger. Dr. Kelman also found that migraineurs who had triggers had more trouble staying asleep, were less likely to rate their sleep as "normal," and also experienced more depression, anxiety, mood swings, and aches and pains than migraineurs who did not have triggers.

The results of a recent study highlight the fact that an association between headache and sleep disturbances is not solely an adult phenomenon. In a presentation given at the Annual Conference on Sleep Disorders in Infants and Childhood in January 2006, pediatric neurologist Kenneth Mack of Mayo Clinic reported that chronic headache in children appears to be linked with sleep disturbances. His team studied 100 children with chronic headache and found that two-thirds of them also had sleep problems (delay in onset of sleep, waking during the night, not feeling refreshed in the morning), and that it was not clear which came first: the headache or the sleep disturbance. The recommendation of the study's authors, however, was to treat both simultaneously. This is, of course, what we do in the Migraine Cure when we recommend specific hormones and supplements to restore balance to various systems that contribute to migraine, and ultimately to balance the sympathetic and parasympathetic nervous systems.

Since we know that sleep disturbances are directly associated with migraine, an effective treatment for these disturbances could conceivably benefit migraine as well. That certainly has been the case with melatonin. So what should you know about this hormone?

The Pineal Gland And Melatonin

If you recall from our discussions in chapters 1 and 2, the pineal gland is a minute but powerful organ that works closely with the hypothalamus to regulate activities that are intimately related to migraine. Let's begin with a look at the hormone that is key to those activities, melatonin.

Melatonin

Melatonin is a hormone produced and secreted by the pineal gland. The manufacturing process begins with tryptophan, an amino acid found in certain foods. The body converts tryptophan into serotonin, a neurotransmitter and hormone that has the ability to regulate pain signals in the brain and can also trigger inflammation of blood vessels in the brain, resulting in migraine pain. The pineal gland then converts the serotonin into melatonin. If the body has a deficiency of tryptophan and/or serotonin, a sufficient amount of melatonin cannot be produced. Stress, including the presence of chronic pain, and poor dietary habits can lead to deficiencies of serotonin and melatonin. In addition, abnormal circadian rhythms of cortisol (the stress hormone) secretion may appear when melatonin levels are low and thus help perpetuate the situation: stress leads to a melatonin deficiency, and insufficient melatonin causes cortisol secretion rhythms to go awry.

This final step in the production process of melatonin occurs only at night. That's because the manufacture and release of melatonin are stimulated by darkness and suppressed by light, which makes melatonin one of the most influential factors in the body's circadian rhythm and thus in the sleep cycle.

Research findings support the idea that since melatonin has a role in synchronizing biological rhythms, and migraine is associated with an imbalance in such rhythms (e.g., hormone imbalances, intestinal flora disturbances, sympathetic/parasympathetic system imbalance), that pineal gland irregularity, and thus melatonin imbalance, is involved in the development of migraine. But melatonin's influence on migraine extends beyond the sleep-wake cycle. For example, the pineal gland releases melatonin to calm or help balance the activity of the endocrine glands (e.g., pituitary, pineal, ovaries, testes, adrenals) when these glands are under stress. Thus if your pituitary releases too much, say, thyroid-stimulating hormone (TSH), when you are under stress, the pineal gland can secrete melatonin to counteract it. Melatonin also has an impact on the levels of estrogen, a key hormone in migraine. Research shows that as the level of follicle-stimulating hormone (FSH; the hormone that stimulates secretion of estrogen) increases, the level of melatonin decreases.

Melatonin and the Sleep Cycle

Now that you have been introduced to melatonin, let's explore its role in the sleep cycle and migraine. The human body has an internal biological "clock" that controls certain circadian (from the latin "circa diem," meaning *about a day*, or *daily*) rhythms. Known as the *suprachiasmatic nucleus*, or SCN, this pinpoint-sized area in the hypothalamus regulates the circadian rhythms of various processes, including the sleep-wake cycle, hormone production, digestive secretions, body temperature, and blood pressure, among others.

All of the circadian rhythms are controlled by internal as well as external, or environmental factors. The most common of the latter type are light and temperature, and it is light we will talk about here. The SCN responds to nature's light and dark—day and night — cycle, which corresponds to the sleep-wake cycle. Briefly, this is how it works.

When light enters the eyes, it activates cells in the retina, which sends signals along the optic nerve to the SCN, which then produces other signals that are sent throughout the body. Some of those signals travel to the pineal gland, telling it that light is present, which causes the gland to shut down its production of melatonin. Levels of melatonin stay low during the daylight hours, but as dusk approaches, the pineal gland receives signals that light is absent. This is also an indication for melatonin production to kick into gear. When the body's level of melatonin increases, the individual becomes drowsy as the body prepares for sleep. Melatonin levels typically peak just before midnight, then gradually decline over the next few hours. As they decline the body gradually wakes up, and the entire cycle begins again.

We already know that migraine has multiple factors that contribute to its development. Therefore although melatonin is an important piece in the migraine and sleep disturbance puzzle, it is not *the* cause of either condition. In fact, it's been shown that people who don't secrete melatonin are still able to sleep. However, restoration of balanced pineal gland function and healthy sleep patterns are critical components in the Migraine Cure treatment program.

Melatonin, Migraine, and Other Head Pain

Clinical evidence that melatonin is not only intimately associated with migraine but also effective in preventing and treating migraine and other types of headache pain is impressive. In a recent study (2004), for example, investigators found that female migraineurs, when compared with healthy controls, had significantly suppressed melatonin levels when exposed to light. Low levels of melatonin in migraine patients suggests supplementation may be beneficial, and that has proven to be true.

For example, in a four-month study of 34 migraine patients (29 women) who had a history of two to eight migraine episodes per month, researchers instructed the individuals to keep a diary for one month and document the details of any migraine activity. Then, beginning with the second month, the individuals took 3 mg of melatonin each night 30 minutes before bedtime. Of the 32 patients who completed the study, eight said their migraines had disappeared, seven reported a 75 percent reduction in migraines, and ten said they had a 50 to 75 percent decrease in migraines. Overall, the intensity of head pain decreased from an average intensity of 7 (on a scale of 0 to 10) at the beginning of the study to just over 3 by the end of the study.

In a Dutch study published in Headache in 1998, the authors found that people with chronic tension headache, migraine, or cluster headache who were taking melatonin to treat a sleep disturbance were completely or almost completely relieved of their head pain within just a few weeks of starting melatonin. One of the study's participants, a fifty-four-year-old man who had suffered with debilitating migraines twice a week for years, had only three migraines during an entire twelve-month period once he started taking melatonin. Three women who had chronic tension-type headache before they entered the study got complete relief from their head pain within two weeks.

Melatonin was also helpful in relieving cluster headache in a group of 20 patients who participated in a double-blind, placebo-controlled study. Fifty percent of the treated patients had no further attacks within three to five days of beginning treatment with melatonin, but the headaches returned when they stopped treatment.

One thing that's important to remember about research that shows the effectiveness of melatonin in eliminating migraine is that the patients in these studies did not completely eliminate their migraine or other head pain because **melatonin was used alone.** To achieve 100 percent elimination of migraine, use of melatonin needs to be **combined** with the other components of our program.

Melatonin, Nitric Oxide, and Migraine

For many years the medical community has known that when heart patients place a nitroglycerin pill under the tongue to prevent angina, the nitroglycerin changes to nitric oxide, a substance that immediately causes the blood vessels in the heart to dilate. Some of these patients, however, also experience a migraine within about six hours of taking the nitroglycerin. This is "a very common side effect," says Jes Olesen, MD, chairman of the neurology department at the University of Copenhagen. "It seems very, very likely that nitric oxide in the brain has some role in triggering migraines—not just in heart patients but in all patients." This finding is echoed by investigators at the Brain Foundation in Australia, who report that nitric oxide "is critical in the development of pain of migraine."

The "critical" element is that people with migraine are hypersensitive to nitric oxide. Indeed, dozens, if not scores of studies have shown that elevated levels of nitric oxide is a cause of migraine pain and chronic tension headache. (You can see an extensive list of these studies at **http://www.neurotransmitter.net/migraineno.html**). So what is nitric oxide?

Nitric oxide is a very simple molecule, composed of one atom of oxygen and one of nitrogen. At one time nitric oxide was believed to have no redeeming value. In fact, it was viewed as an environmental pollutant: nitric oxide is emitted into the air through the exhaust pipes of gas-run vehicles, where it reacts with oxygen to produce smog. Then researchers discovered that it is indeed important to human health. Specifically, the endothelial cells that line the walls of blood vessels synthesize nitric oxide to relax the muscles, which in turn dilate the blood vessels and increase blood flow. The molecule has a very short life-span, and so the endothelial cells manufacture a constant supply in response to the stress of the blood flow on the vessel walls.

When blood vessels are constricted and need to be dilated—widened—as when someone is having an angina attack, then nitric oxide is helpful. But when someone is hypersensitive to elevated levels of nitric oxide and their blood vessels arbitrarily dilate and cause excessive pressure, then nitric oxide is problematic. For some migraineurs, nitric oxide could be a contributing factor in their pain.

Nitric oxide also is a neurotransmitter, which means it has the ability to transmit signals between neurons, including those in the brain in the head and in the "second brain," the gut, where it can decrease the spasms in the muscles of the gastrointestinal tract. Therefore, you can see that nitric oxide plays a role in at least two components of the Migraine Cure: pineal gland restoration, and in the digestive tract, which we discuss in chapter 6.

Experts in the pharmaceutical industry have looked eagerly at the emerging information about nitric oxide and migraine and turned their eyes toward the development of drugs which, in the words of investigators at the Brain Foundation in Australia, are "targeted at nitric oxide . . . [and] may prove to be better and more specific than the anti-migraine drugs currently in use." Rather than drugs, however, we may turn to a natural approach, a component of the Migraine Cure, melatonin.

According to a report in *Medical Hypotheses* (January 2006), nitric oxide is released toward the end of the sleep cycle. Stress, disrupted sleep, and loss of sleep continuity, which are accompanied by an increase in the stress hormone, cortisol, are all associated with an increase in the amount and duration of nitric oxide released at night. Melatonin, as you've learned, not only helps promote sleep and prevent migraine, it also inhibits production of excess nitric oxide. Therefore this is yet another reason why melatonin is an important addition to the Migraine Cure.

Melatonin and High Blood Pressure

It's been shown that migraineurs with aura are 76 percent more likely to have high blood pressure (hypertension). This increased risk of high blood pressure is a major concern, so evidence that melatonin is effective in reducing both systolic and diastolic blood pressure is good news for migraineurs. So far several studies support this. In a double-blind, placebo-controlled study, sixteen men who had untreated hypertension took 2.5 mg of melatonin one hour before bedtime for three weeks and experienced, on average, a six-point decline in systolic blood pressure and a four-point drop in diastolic pressure. In another double-blind, placebo-controlled trial, this one in eighteen women, a three-week course of 3 mg of melatonin significantly reduced nighttime blood pressure.

Taking Melatonin

Melatonin supplements are widely available, from grocery stores to pharmacies, health food stores, mail order, and department stores. As part of the pineal restoration segment of the Migraine Cure, I recommend a combination product that contains melatonin (3 mg), vitamin B6, and kava kava, one or two capsules taken at bedtime, depending on the individual's needs. (I discuss the merits of vitamin B6 and kava kava below.) Suzanne, for example, had been a migraineur for about twelve years when she first contacted us. Her migraines had started at age twenty and came at a rate of about two to four per month. Along with migraine, her other major symptoms included relentless fatigue, insomnia, and lack of sex drive. During her first month on the program, which included hormone restoration, probiotics, magnesium, and a melatonin combination supplement, Suzanne had no migraines, and she said "I definitely have much more energy and my sex drive is beginning to return."

Suzanne's insomnia, however, had not responded to the melatonin, so we increased her dose from one to two capsules (6 mg) before bedtime. Within a few days her insomnia resolved, and over the next two months she was able to decrease the dose to one capsule. By the end of another two months her sleep patterns were normal, so she stopped taking melatonin.

Today Suzanne is migraine- and insomnia-free and has only taken melatonin once in the last two months.

In most cases, patients only need to take melatonin for a few months, until the pineal circadian cycle is restored. Then they may take it periodically for a few days per month or every few months if their sleep becomes disturbed. Side effects of melatonin, which are rare, may include morning grogginess, undesired drowsiness, and disorientation. These problems usually do not occur if you take melatonin as directed and typically disappear once the dose is reduced.

Melatonin, IBS, and Other Migraine-Related Symptoms

In chapter 6, I talk about the intimate link between gastrointestinal disorders and migraine, but here I want to preview that discussion by noting another connection: how supplementation with melatonin can improve abdominal pain in people who have sleep disturbances and irritable bowel syndrome. This relationship has been reported in several studies and is yet one more example of how seemingly diverse and separate components of the Migraine Cure are linked together. The association also highlights the importance of restoring balance to several critical and related systems in the body in the quest to eliminate migraine.

In one of the studies, a double-blind, placebo-controlled trial, seventeen women with irritable bowel syndrome received either 3 mg of melatonin or placebo for eight weeks, nothing for four weeks, and then either melatonin or placebo again. Symptoms of irritable bowel were significantly improved when the women were taking melatonin, but not when they were taking a placebo.

Another benefit of melatonin appears to be for patients who have fibromyalgia. (Note: In chapter 8 you can read about Priscilla, a woman who had fibromyalgia, migraine, sleep disturbances, and many other complaints and how she responded to the migraine treatment program.) In a study designed to determine the possible effects of melatonin on symptoms of fibromyalgia, including sleep disturbances, fatigue, depression, and pain, 21 patients with fibromyalgia participated in a four-week pilot study in which they took 3 mg of melatonin at bedtime each night. Of the nineteen patients who completed the study, all reported significant improvement in sleep and severity of pain at selected tender points.

Yet another study looked at the effect of melatonin on perimenopausal and menopausal women. The women, ages 42 to 62 years, took 3 mg of melatonin or a placebo for six months and had their hormone levels checked from saliva and blood samples throughout the study. The researchers found that melatonin helped shift sex hormone levels back toward optimal ranges, improved thyroid function, and eliminated depression related to menopause.

Kava Kava

In addition to melatonin, we recommend kava kava as part of the restoration program for pineal function. Kava kava is an herb that was widely used in Europe and many countries around the world as a natural tranquilizer and treatment for anxiety. It has been highly respected for centuries by inhabitants of the Polynesian islands and New Guinea, where this member of the pepper family is primarily found. Kava root extract, which is derived from the root of *Piper methysticum*, has a calming effect, promotes sleep, and relaxes deep muscles, abilities attributed to components called kavalactones. Kava also has a mild calcium channel blocker effect in that is can reduce excitability of the cell membranes. Calcium channel blockers, as I mentioned in chapter 3, are sometimes prescribed for migraine. When you use kava kava, you have the benefits of calcium channel blocking drugs without the side effects.

Is Kava Kava Safe?

Before 2002, kava extracts were used widely and extensively throughout Europe and other countries and were viewed as a safe, effective treatment for daily use. Side effects, which are rare and typically seen only with excessive, long-term use, may include scaly yellowing of the skin, yellowing of the nails or hair, eye irritation, tiredness, or impaired motor reflexes. These disappear once the herb is stopped. Near the end of 2002, however, a single study conducted in Germany suggested the herb may cause liver damage, including hepatitis, liver failure, and cirrhosis. By January 2003, use of kava was banned in the entire European Union and Canada, but it is still allowed to be marketed in the United States, along with warnings about possible liver damage. All of these actions were taken based on the results of one study. Subsequent reviews and analyses of specific clinical trials from around the world, however, have revealed several critical facts that were not reported along with the damaging study. Namely:

> • Most of the people who reported side effects were taking more than ten times the recommended daily dose of kava (4,000 to 10,000 mg). A typical dose is 100 to 500 mg taken 30 minutes before bedtime. As with any substance, taking kava in extremely high doses can potentially cause adverse effects.
> • Most of the people who had liver problems were taking at least one other prescription medication along with kava, which increases the possibility that the medication(s) were responsible for the liver damage.
> • Many of the people with liver damage also consumed alcohol regularly, and alcohol alone is known to cause liver damage.
> • This point could be a coincidence, but when the study results were released, a drug company was trying to launch a new antidepressant.

What the Research Shows

It's important to emphasize that both before but more importantly after the release of this one damaging report, there have been many other studies in which kava has been found to be an effective and safe for treatment of anxiety.

A 2004 study, for example, found that kava extract safely and effectively provided relief for patients who had sleep disturbances associated with anxiety. In Germany, researchers conducted a double-blind, placebo-controlled study of 58 patients who had anxiety syndrome. The treated patients received 100 mg of kava extract three times daily for four weeks. After only one week, individuals who had taken kava had a significant reduction in their anxiety symptoms compared with patients who had taken a placebo, and they continued to improve throughout the study. Similar results were found in another German study in which 50 patients received 50 mg three times daily for four weeks.

One of the most telling reports is a meta-analysis in which investigators evaluated eleven trials that included a total of 645 participants. Compared with placebo, kava extract was found to be an effective treatment for anxiety and to be relatively safe for up to six months. Two other interesting trials looked at the use of kava and hormone replacement therapy in postmenopausal women and their effect on anxiety and depression. The study showed that this combination was "an excellent therapeutic tool" for postmenopausal women, "in particular those suffering from anxiety and depression."

My experience has been that if you take kava responsibly in clinically tested doses, the supplement is very safe. Patients who follow the Migraine Cure plan as recommended typically take melatonin and kava at the beginning of the program, but once they are migraine-free—which usually happens within two to four weeks—they can reduce their use of melatonin and kava to a minimal dose and discontinue them later, depending on how well their sleep problems have resolved. At the same time, we always recommend that individuals have blood tests periodically to check their hormone levels and liver and kidney functions, so there is always a check-and-balance system in place to monitor your progress as well as alert you to any changes you may need to make to your program.

Vitamin B6

Vitamin B6 (pyridoxine) is an important part of the migraine treatment program for several reasons. When it comes to restoring pineal function, vitamin B6 is necessary for the production of serotonin, the brain neurotransmitter that has a major role in the sleep-wake cycle, chronic pain, mood, and appetite. I also recommend it because, like kava kava, it has a calming effect. The typical dose is 10 to 20 mg taken 30 minutes before bedtime.

> Vitamin B6 also plays other essential roles in the body that are important in the prevention and elimination of migraine; namely, it:
> - Promotes healthy digestion.
> - Aids in proper nutrition, as it helps break down of protein, carbohydrates, and fats, which is necessary for proper utilization of nutrients from food.
> - Helps prevent fatigue by releasing carbohydrates that are stored as energy in the muscles and liver.
> - Helps relieve symptoms of premenstrual syndrome.
> - Enhances immune system activity and thus helps the body better withstand stress. Along with the other B complex vitamins, pyridoxine is viewed as an "anti-stress" vitamin.

Certain conditions can increase your need for vitamin B6, including several that are commonly associated with migraine, such as stress, diarrhea, long-term illness, and intestinal problems. In some individuals, a deficiency of vitamin B6 can occur and result in insomnia, depression, nervousness, weakness, rash, anemia, cracked lips, or irritability.

In Conclusion

To restore optimal function to the pineal gland, I recommend supplementation with melatonin (3 to 6 mg), kava root extract (250 to 500 mg), and vitamin B6 (10 to 20 mg), taken about 30 minutes before bedtime, with adjustments made to dosages to meet your specific needs. Depending on your response to these supplements and to the other components of the program, you may need to take this combination of supplements for only a month or two. Then, once your pineal gland has reset itself and is functioning well, you may take this supplement mix only when you experience sleep disturbance or feel especially anxious.

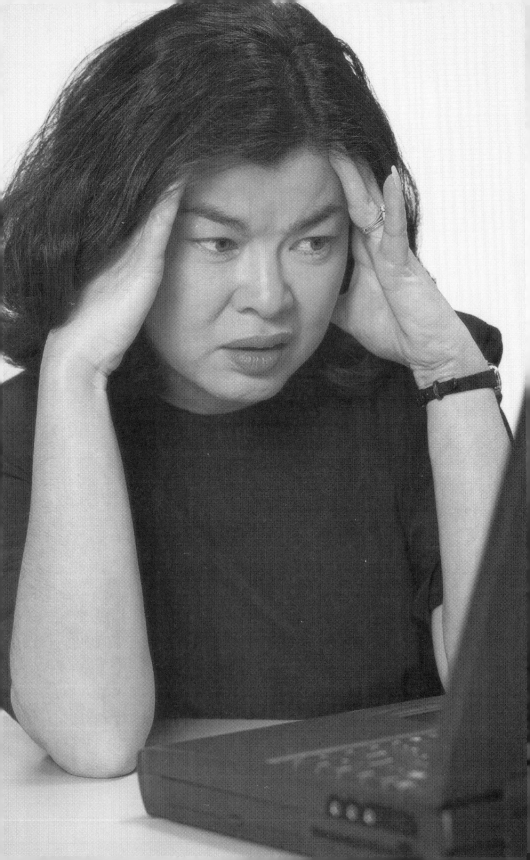

6

Achieving Metabolic Balance

You've probably heard the expression, "the way to a man's heart is through his stomach," but have you ever heard "the way to eliminate your headache is through your gut"? Well, crazy as it sounds, there's a lot of truth in this statement: the link between migraine and gastrointestinal (GI) disorders, and especially the gut (intestinal tract) has been confirmed by numerous studies and clinical observations. Indeed, my own experience has shown me that this brain-and-GI tract connection plays a major role in migraine. It is yet one more example of the fact that migraine is not a single disorder but a collection of disorders, and why I address it as part of the Migraine Cure. That part includes the relationship between your brain— and migraine — and your GI tract, and how to restore balance to this important alliance.

One indication of this critical alliance, just to give you one example, is the fact that most people with migraine also experience constipation. Time and time again, migraineurs have told me how they've been constipated for ten, twenty, even thirty years or longer. Constipation is a symptom that reflects an abnormal intestinal environment—or abnormal *intestinal flora*, a term you will see often — and a sign of an imbalance between the sympathetic and parasympathetic nervous systems. When we restore the health of the gut, we also eliminate constipation, improve absorption of nutrients, balance the digestive system, help restore balance between the sympathetic and parasympathetic systems, and contribute to the elimination of migraine.

In this chapter we will eavesdrop on the "conversations" between the brain and the gut—the nervous and digestive systems — and learn how the messages they exchange impact the development and elimination of migraine. More important, you will learn what you can do to restore balance to your digestive system and thus contribute to the end of your migraine.

The Scene Of The "Crime": The Gut

The often heard expression "you are what you eat" is only partially accurate. In reality, you are what your gut absorbs. This difference in emphasis is especially important in today's world, because so much of the food both in the supermarkets and served in restaurants is contaminated and/or deficient in important nutrients. Therefore on the one hand you are exposed to substances you don't want to absorb, such as pesticides, artificial flavorings and colorings, preservatives, hormones, steroids, heavy metals, antibiotics, and industrial toxins; and on the other hand you have foods that have been refined, processed, and stripped of health-enhancing ingredients. The gut is the center of your food processing activity, and it's also a key player in whether you experience migraine. When the gut is consistently exposed to toxic substances and deprived of essential nutrients, your digestive enzymes are inactivated, your intestinal tract weakens, digestion and nutrient absorption are compromised, and your overall health suffers.

Successful elimination of migraine depends on a healthy gut, and fortunately you have a great deal of control over that environment. One of the most important things you can do to ensure a healthy intestinal tract is maintain a balance between the friendly and unfriendly bacteria—the intestinal flora — that live in the gut. Friendly bacteria are those that provide health-promoting or health-maintaining properties while the unfriendly varieties can impose significant harm to your health. Together, more than four hundred different kinds of intestinal flora live in your bowel.

A healthy, well-functioning gut contains at least 85 percent friendly bacteria and not more than 15 percent unfriendly bacteria. That balance can be upset by various factors, such as:

- Use of pain killers (including nonsteroidal anti-inflammatory drugs) and/or other medications. If you are like most migraineurs, you are taking at least one and more than likely two or more over-the-counter and/or prescription medications related to your migraine (see "Henri's Story" below). You also need to consider medications you may be taking for other medical conditions, such as insomnia, depression, fibromyalgia, arthritis, heart disease, diabetes, irritable bowel, or other gastrointestinal disorders, all of which are common in people who have migraine. Use of these drugs, especially long-term use, can damage the intestinal wall, cause an imbalance in intestinal flora, and jeopardize the absorption of nutrients.
- Diarrhea caused by harmful bacteria or viruses. Most people experience occasional episodes of diarrhea, but among some migraineurs it is frequently chronic and alternates with bouts of constipation.
- Use of antibiotics. This factor alone can have a devastating impact on the health of your intestinal tract and thus your susceptibility to migraine. Although antibiotics typically destroy bad bacteria, they unfortunately also destroy friendly species as well, which disrupts the balance between these two types of organisms. Antibiotics also promote the development of resistant bacteria in the intestinal tract, and these damaging bacteria can result in infections in other parts of the body.
- Surgical procedures performed on the bowel.
- A unhealthy diet, one that consists of processed and refined foods, simple sugars, soft drinks, alcohol, fried foods, and items that contain pesticides, hormones, steroids, antibiotics, and preservatives.
- Emotional stress. While emotional stress alone does not directly cause gastrointestinal disorders, it does worsen symptoms.
- Conditions that cause abnormal functioning of the bowel (e.g., Crohn's disease, ulcerative colitis, irritable bowel syndrome.)
- Exposure to chemotherapy and/or radiotherapy.

Henri's Story

Henri is a thirty-two-year-old fast-food restaurant manager who had been experiencing migraine headaches roughly every other day for nearly fifteen years when he first talked to us. At five-foot-eight and 182 pounds, he confessed that he didn't get much exercise, mostly because he was "too fatigued" most of the time. He also had a history of seasonal allergies since adolescence, and for the last ten years or so he had increasingly been bothered by insomnia and other sleep disturbances, depression, anxiety, and irritable bowel syndrome.

Although migraine was Henri's main complaint, he was also especially disturbed by alternating bouts of constipation and diarrhea, which he said were making it difficult to work. He didn't smoke, but he did like to have an occasional beer, even though he thought the alcohol "might, but it's hard to tell" trigger migraine. At one time he had taken sumatriptan for about six months to prevent migraine, but because he didn't have insurance at the time, and currently did not have adequate coverage, he said it was too expensive to continue. Since then he had been treating the symptoms, including his gastrointestinal problems, with over-the-counter medications, including nonsteroidal anti-inflammatory drugs (NSAIDs) and loperamide (Imodium®), which he took almost daily.

After we spoke at length with Henri in January 2005, we recommended he undergo a lipid panel and hormone panel. His results were as follows:

- Total cholesterol: 224 mmHg (<200 mmHg)
- DHEA-S: 116 ug/dL (280-640 ug/dL)
- Pregnenolone: <10 ng/dL (10-200 ng/dL)
- Estradiol: 11 pg/mL (0-53 pg/mL)
- Progesterone: 0.5 ng/mL (0.3-1.2 ng/mL)
- Testosterone: 511 ng/dL (241-827 ng/dL)

Based on the results and Henri's symptoms, we recommended the following:

- DHEA: 100 mg in the morning
- 7-keto: 100 mg in the morning
- Pregnenolone: 300 mg in the morning
- Saw palmetto: 160 mg in the morning
- Zinc: 30 mg in the morning
- Magnesium citrate: Powdered supplement, each dose (1 scoop) contains 420 mg of magnesium citrate. Recommended dose for Henri was 1/3 scoop in the morning and one scoop in the evening.
- Melatonin formula: each capsule contains 3 mg of melatonin, 250 mg of kava root extract, and 10 mg of vitamin B6. Henri's recommended dose was one capsule at bedtime.
- Probiotic formula: Contains 3.5 billion *Lactobacillus* group (*L. rhamnosus A, L. rhamnosus B, L. acidophilus, L. casei, L. bulgaricus*), 1.0 billion *Bifidobacterium* group (*B. longum, B. breve*), and 0.5 billion *Streptococcus thermophilus*. It also contains gluten-free grasses, algae, natural fiber, herbs, and bioflavonoid extracts. One scoop in the morning. After one month, he added one scoop in the evening.
- Progesterone: 1/2 tsp cream at night to promote sleep through additional stimulation of the parasympathetic nervous system.

Henri reported back after he had been on the program for one month and noted he had had only one headache, "but it definitely wasn't a migraine," he said. "It was related to my allergies. And I think I got it because I had decided to go cold turkey—I stopped taking all the meds I was taking for migraine and my allergies. But, hey, just one allergy headache in one month is incredible. I can't believe it."

Henri was still having significant problems with his irritable bowel symptoms, however, and he was very reluctant to stop taking his medications for them. We felt he needed to increase his use of probiotics, given his long history of medication use, so we suggested he add one more scoop in the evening before bedtime. He called us again in March 2005 and said his irritable bowel was completely gone and that he was no longer taking the loperamide. In addition, he said his mood had improved "one thousand percent," and that he had lots of energy. We suggested he get another blood test so we could monitor his hormone levels, but he chose not to do so, and we did not hear back from him again.

When the balance tips in favor of the bad bacteria, the gut becomes damaged and inflamed. This condition, often called dysbiosis, is characterized by symptoms such as diarrhea, constipation, gas, abdominal pain, cramping, and bloating. More important, the toxins from these bad bacteria can enter the bloodstream, infiltrate your tissues, and result in conditions such as migraine, arthritis, fibromyalgia, chronic fatigue, and depression. Inflammation in the gut damages the proteins that are needed to transport minerals from the intestines to the blood, and the result can be a variety of nutritional deficiencies and their consequences.

For example, a deficiency of magnesium—a nutrient that plays a major role in migraine and is discussed in detail in chapter 7—is common in individuals who have migraine and in those who have fibromyalgia. Magnesium supplementation can keep the blood vessels healthy and promote good blood flow, which helps prevent migraine, while the mineral can eliminate the muscle pain and spasms characteristic of fibromyalgia. However, magnesium supplements will be ineffective in people who have these conditions if they do not restore and maintain the health of their intestinal flora. Again, you can see that it is important to restore balance to more than one system in order to eliminate migraine.

The Brain-Gut Axis

Do you get butterflies in your stomach when you have to give a speech? Have you ever done something on "gut instinct" or because it felt right "in your gut"? These pat or colloquial phrases draw attention to a very real phenomenon, a network characterized by a continuous, busy exchange of electrical and chemical signals that takes place between the central nervous system (brain) and the digestive system (gut), a network experts have dubbed the *brain-gut axis*. Some scientists have even called the gut the "second brain," and this concept is not farfetched for several important, and scientifically proven, reasons.

One is that many of the vital components found in the brain are also found in the gut, including neurotransmitters (serotonin—95 percent of the serotonin in the body resides in the gut; also dopamine, norepinephrine, and nitric oxide), various brain proteins, and enkephalins (one of the body's natural painkillers). Another is the influence of stress on the occurrence and severity of symptoms is associated with hyperactivity of the HPA axis which, as we discussed in chapter 2, is controlled by the brain. Yet another is the presence and function of the physical connection between these two brains, the vagus nerve.

The Vagus Nerve Highway

The vagus nerve is one of the longest nerves in the body. It runs from the brain stem through organs in the neck, thorax, and abdomen and is a major transportation pathway for chemical and electrical signals that pass between the brain and gut. And there is a lot of traffic on this pathway. The brain, for example, releases acetylcholine and adrenaline, which signal the stomach when to produce acid and when to stop, and also sends messages to the intestines about when to move along its contents. In return, the digestive system responds by sending signals to the brain that result in such sensations as nausea, pain, hunger, and fullness. Stress signals from the brain can also change nerve function between the gut and the esophagus and cause heartburn.

Some of the signals sent from the gut can also affect mood. Messages that travel from the gut to the brain reach the limbic system, an area of the brain stem that affects mood, sleep, and appetite, among other things. In fact, scientists capitalized on this information to develop a new treatment technique for depression. Called vagus nerve stimulation therapy, or VNS, it involves implanting a tiny device in the left chest that generates mild electrical impulses that stimulate the vagus nerve. Studies show that VNS, which was approved for use in depression in 2005 by the Food and Drug

Administration, can relieve depression and cause feelings of well-being. It is believed this occurs because the electrical impulses alter the levels of certain neurotransmitters, including serotonin, brain chemicals that play a major role in emotions and in migraine.

Gastrointestinal Disorders and Migraine

When we consider that 95 percent of the serotonin in the body is in the digestive system and that 95 percent of the fibers in the vagus nerve run from the gut to the brain, there appears to be a lot of potential for "feelings" to travel between the gut and the brain, and many opportunities for emotions to contribute to imbalances in hormone levels and, perhaps more important, the intestinal flora. Here are a few examples.

I have already mentioned that constipation and migraine often go hand-in-hand, but it is by no means the only gut-brain/migraine relationship. Seventy percent of migraineurs have some type of gastrointestinal disorder as part of their disease syndrome. Fear and stress, for example, stimulate the vagus nerve to increase serotonin activity in the gut. This activity in turn overstimulates the gut and diarrhea is the result. Indeed, many migraineurs also experience irritable bowel syndrome, Crohn's disease, or ulcerative colitis which, along with constipation and diarrhea, are all conditions associated with, but not caused by, stress. That is, emotional stress alone does not cause irritable bowel and other GI disorders, but it can worsen their symptoms.

One recent study, in fact, found that chronic distress was responsible for 97 percent of all changes in irritable bowel syndrome symptoms. What happens is this: when you experience stress, your body produces adrenaline and corticotrophin-releasing factor (which causes the release of cortisol, the stress hormone). Frequent or chronic stress causes these substances to be released at levels that can attack your digestive system, cause diarrhea or constipation, and cause the cells in the gut to be hypersensitive to pain.

The Gut, The Brain, and Sleep

The brain and the gut influence each other when it comes to sleep as well. According to Dr. David Wingate, a professor of gastrointestinal science at the University of London, during sleep the brain produces 90-minute cycles of slow-wave sleep accompanied by rapid eye movement (REM) sleep. Similarly, during the night, when you are fasting, the gut's brain produces 90-minute cycles of slow-wave muscle contractions accompanied by brief bursts of rapid muscle movements. What are the results of these "conversations" between the two brains? Individuals who have migraine and GI problems often have sleep difficulties as well, including abnormal REM sleep. And who hasn't blamed a pepperoni pizza or other stomach-irritating food for nightmares experienced later that evening, evidence that indigestion can affect brain activity and hence our dreams.

The Melatonin-GI Connection

Sometimes it seems as if there is always a new relationship being uncovered between different components of the Migraine Cure that further support why it works. Case in point is a recent (2005) double-blind, placebo-controlled study that showed how melatonin improved symptoms of irritable bowel syndrome (IBS) (abdominal pain, rectal urgency, sensitivity to pain) in individuals who suffered with sleep disturbance along with the IBS.

The forty patients in the two-week study were divided into two groups: twenty received 3 mg of melatonin daily at bedtime, and twenty received placebo. At the end of the two weeks, the patients who had taken melatonin reported 58 percent less abdominal pain compared with 18 percent in the placebo group. The treated patients also reported an improvement in pain and rectal urgency, but the placebo group did not.

The Brain-Gut Axis: Bottom Line

As a person with migraine, when your gut feels like it is in knots—when you have symptoms of diarrhea, constipation, irritable bowel, or abdominal pain—you need to restore balance to your intestinal flora if you want to rid yourself not only of your gut pain but your migraine as well. I found an excellent way to accomplish this goal is through supplementation with probiotics.

How To Restore Balance: Probiotics

Probiotics are supplements of live, friendly bacteria that you can take to enhance or restore the balance of bacterial flora in your intestinal tract. The most common and essential of the friendly bacteria are the *Bifidobacteria*, *Streptococcus*, and *Lactobacilli* species, which perform many functions essential for health and well-being. For example, they can:

- Assist in the absorption of nutrients into the bloodstream.
- Form a barrier against harmful bacteria that can cause diarrhea.
- Manufacture food for your intestinal cells so they can function optimally.
- Some produce natural antibiotics that destroy harmful bacteria, viruses, yeasts, and fungi.
- Help prevent harmful bacteria from causing damage.
- Prevent symptoms caused by use of antibiotics, which can destroy the majority of the friendly bacteria in the intestinal tract.

Using Probiotics

When it comes to buying probiotics, it's a "buyer beware" market because, unlike drugs, nutritional supplements are not regulated by the Food and Drug Administration. As a consumer you need to do your homework and buy your supplements only from reputable manufacturers. After much research and experimentation, the probiotic supplement I recommend is a powdered formula that contains 3.5 billion of *Lactobacillus* group (*L. rhamnosus A, L. rhamnosus B* [these two species are sometimes referred to as *Lactobacillus GG*], *L. acidophilus, L. casei, L. bulgaricus*), 1 billion of *Bifidobacterium* group (*B. longum, B. breve*), and 0.5 billion of *Streptococcus thermophilus* per dose (see Appendix for product information). It is well tolerated, easy to use, and has helped a great many people.

One of those people is Connie, a fifty-five-year-old former retail store manager whose main complaints were migraine, fibromyalgia, constipation, back and neck pain, depression, and sleep disturbances when she first sought help from us in early 2002. You can read Connie's complete story in chapter 9, but here I want to highlight how we met the challenge she had with constipation.

Four weeks after Connie started taking the bio-identical hormones, pineal restoration supplement, and probiotics we recommended for her, she contacted us and told us how excited she was that her migraines were nearly gone and that her depression, pain, and sleep had improved. Constipation, however, was still a significant problem, even though she was taking the recommended one scoop of probiotic formula every day. Because Connie had a long history of prescription and over-the-counter drug use that matched her long list of medical conditions, we suspected her intestinal flora was greatly compromised from years of assault. Therefore we suggested she add two scoops of the magnesium citrate supplement to her daily program, plus increase her probiotic supplement to two scoops per day. As additional support, we also suggested she significantly reduce her use of dietary sugar and that she use a one-month parasite-cleansing program that contains a mixture of herbs, fiber, and fructooligosaccharides (FOS). FOS are nondigestible fibers that support and promote friendly bacteria in the gut, and they are often recommended for people who have irritable bowel syndrome and other gastrointestinal disorders. Within the month her constipation disappeared completely, and she also continued to improve in other areas as well.

If you choose to use a different probiotic than the one recommended, please consider the following guidelines when making your purchase.

- Viability count. This is the number of live organisms in the product. Independent testing laboratories have found that some products do not come close to the number they claim on the label. You can contact an independent testing laboratory, like Consumer Labs (www.ConsumerLab.com), which tests and reports on nutritional supplements, for reliable brands.

> - Probiotics should be refrigerated to ensure their potency and viability.
> - Make sure the product label lists the genus and species (in italics), and preferably the strain as well—for example, *Lactobacillus plantarum* ST31. Generally, stating a strain indicates that the manufacturer has made a commitment to standardize their product. The strain may be displayed as numbers or letters.

Probiotics and Food Triggers

We have already established that the majority of migraineurs have at least one trigger that can set off a migraine attack, and among those triggers are various foods and beverages. It's also known that diet plays a significant role in precipitating migraine in children and adolescents. The exact prevalence of food allergies among children or adults, with or without migraine, is uncertain and a point of debate. It's been reported that approximately 15 percent of children born in Western countries have a least one type of food allergy, and that an estimated 20 percent of the population in the same countries suffer with atopic (allergy) diseases, which include food allergies. Unfortunately, although food triggers are common among migraineurs, there are very few studies of the relationship between food allergies and migraine and/or headache.

There are studies, however, showing that use of probiotics can prevent the development of food allergies and relieve the related symptoms. These benefits may be the result of the ability of probiotics to improve digestion, help the gut control the absorption of food allergens, or alter how the immune system responds to the allergens. Two studies in which lactobacillus GG bacteria *(L. rhamnosus* A and *L. rhamnosus* B) were given to infants with food allergies found probiotics to be useful in the treatment of these children. I have no reason to believe that probiotics would not be beneficial in preventing food triggers and allergies in adults and/or migraineurs as well.

Supporting Digestive Health

Use of probiotics is the cornerstone of the restoration of intestinal flora in the Migraine Cure, but there are also other steps you can consider. Personally I find that most people who have suffered with migraine for many years have long been prevented from enjoying some of life's pleasures, and for many people that includes foods and beverages they have had to avoid because they triggered migraine. Therefore, although I certainly advocate eating a nutritious diet, I normally don't introduce any dietary instructions as part of the Migraine Cure. I prefer to let individuals establish some normalcy in their lives, and then some of them discover that because they feel so good, they want to make positive lifestyle changes, whether it be switching to organic foods, starting an exercise program, or participating in stress reduction techniques.

Given that introduction, there are some steps you can take to further support and promote your digestive health. I discuss them briefly here.

Dietary Help

Some patients ask whether they should follow a specific type of diet to help balance their intestinal flora and enhance the overall treatment process as well. Certainly a well-balanced, nutritionally rich, whole foods diet is an excellent choice for everyone, including people who have migraine. A diet that includes refined and processed foods, simple sugars, fried foods, partially hydrogenated fats, and foods that have been treated with pesticides, hormones, steroids, and/or antibiotics places a great deal of stress on the digestive system as it tries to process the chemicals and other toxins. In particular, if you eat meat, your better choice is hormone-free products to avoid the added influence of hormones. In addition, I encourage patients to enjoy whole foods as much as possible, including fresh fruits and vegetables, whole grains, fish (focus on small, cold-water fish such as sardines, herring, some salmon), nuts, seeds, and beans.

Prebiotics

Prebiotics are substances that nourish and support the friendly bacteria that live in your intestinal tract and help prevent infection. Most prebiotics are oligosaccharides, a type of short-chain sugar molecule. Examples of oligosaccharides include fructooligosaccharides (FOS), galactooligosaccharides (GOS), and inulin, which is a type of fructose oligosaccharide. When you eat these substances, your body does not digest them completely, and the undigested part is used to nourish the friendly bacteria (especially *Bifidobacteria* and *Lactobacillus*) in your gut. These prebiotics also help increase the number of friendly bacteria and reduce the amount of damaging bacteria. Some studies also suggest FOS or inulin may help reduce elevated cholesterol and triglyceride levels, but results are inconsistent.

FOS, GOS, and inulin are available as supplements in tablets, capsules, and as a powder. (The probiotic mixture that we recommend as part of the Migraine Cure contains FOS.) FOS and inulin can also be found in onions, leeks, asparagus, Jerusalem artichokes, and chicory. Soybeans are one of the main sources of GOS, which can be synthesized from milk sugar (lactose).

If You Need a Laxative

People who have followed the migraine program typically experience complete elimination of constipation, diarrhea, and irritable bowel problems, some within a week or two, others within a month or longer. To normalize bowel movements and to correct any digestive problems, we always prefer that individuals use a natural approach rather than resort to use of laxatives. That approach, as you've seen, involves restoring normal function of the parasympathetic nervous system at night by using extra doses of progesterone, magnesium, and melatonin. We can also make adjustments to the probiotic dosage and/or suggest additional supplements, such as multiple digestive enzymes.

That being said, if you follow our program and find you consistently need a laxative, consult with your physician as soon as possible so he or she can do a diagnostic workup to rule out any serious reason for your constipation. If you find that you occasionally need a laxative, you want to use a product that ensures the health of your intestinal flora, which means steer clear of synthetic commercial products and reach for natural herbal laxatives.

Laxatives come in four different types. Stimulant laxatives increase contractions in the intestinal tract, osmotic agents soften the stools by increasing their water content, lubricants ease elimination, and bulk-forming products increase the volume of the intestinal tract and thus stimulate intestinal contractions. Of the four, I recommend the latter, as they are virtually side-effect free (abdominal cramps are a rare occurrence) and do not irritate the intestinal tract, problems you may encounter with use of the other types. Stimulant laxatives, for example, often cause abdominal pain that can be severe. The downside of bulking agents is that they take longer (at least a day or two) than stimulants (the fastest acting), lubricants, and osmotic agents to be effective.

Natural bulking agents contain celluloses, hemicelluloses, lignins, and pectins that resist human digestive enzymes so they pass unchanged through the small intestines into the colon, where resident bacteria break them down. The bacteria also grow on the bulking agents, which results in an increase in stool volume. Because intestinal bacteria flora are key in this process, it is important to maintain as healthy a gut as possible, which you can do by taking probiotics. If you take a bulking agent, drink plenty of liquids, at least five to ten times the dry weight of the product you take. Do not use bulking agents before lying down or before going to bed.

Linseed (flaxseed) is a bulk laxative that contains the dried, ripe seeds of flax. The main components include fatty oil (40-70%), protein (23%), and mucilages (7-12%). Linseed should be taken as crushed seeds, not just the oil, which is ineffective alone. Crushed linseeds can be added to food (two teaspoons taken 2 to 3 times daily for constipation) to make them more palatable. Psyllium, which is derived from the dried ripe seeds of European plantain, acts in a similar way.

In Conclusion

When you want to eliminate migraine, you need to ensure the healthy functioning of not only the brain in your head, but also the health of your second "brain," the one in your gut. As that fact became increasingly obvious to me during my research and clinical observations, addressing that need was made a part of the Migraine Cure. To restore harmony to the intestinal flora, I found that the addition of selected probiotics was most beneficial. After several months of taking this supplement on a daily basis, most people find that occasional use, perhaps once a month, is sufficient to maintain a healthy gut and, as a "bonus," contributes to overall health and well-being.

7

The Ion Balancing Act

This is a short chapter, but don't let its brevity fool you: the step I discuss is critical for the success of the Migraine Cure. And that step is the restoration of the balance between two minerals, ionized magnesium and ionized calcium. The precarious balance between these two elements is intimately connected with the activity of the steroid hormones, the function of the pineal gland, proper functioning of the digestive system, and, by extension, balance between the sympathetic and parasympathetic nervous systems.

First, let me explain what I mean by ionized. An "ion" is an atom or group of atoms that has acquired a positive or negative charge as the result of gaining or losing one or more electrons. Magnesium and calcium can exist in the body either (a) as a freely circulating, active ion—an atom or group of atoms that has acquired a positive or negative charge as the result of gaining or losing one or more electrons; or (b) bound to proteins or other substances. Magnesium and calcium that are ionized are metabolically active and excitable, always seeking something to which they can attach so they can replace their missing electron(s). These ions are free to participate in a wide variety of biochemical body processes and thus can have a tremendous impact on functions in the body. (**Note: When I refer to the calcium/magnesium ratio, I am talking about the ionized forms of these minerals.**)

In this chapter I share with you the importance of the relationship between the calcium/magnesium ratio and migraine, why restoring the balance of this ratio is a key element in the Migraine Cure, and how you can achieve it using one simple supplement. The relationship between this ratio and migraine is not only interesting, it raises some questions as well. What's so special about magnesium that it plays such a big role in migraine? What's going on between ionized magnesium and ionized calcium that causes migraine? What is the relationship between this ratio and the other elements of the Migraine Cure? Let's look at these and other questions.

Magnesium

Magnesium is the fourth most abundant mineral in the human body. At least 50 percent of magnesium is present in bone, while all but 1 percent of the remaining magnesium is found inside the cells of tissues and organs. That 1 percent is found in the bloodstream.

More than three hundred biochemical reactions depend on magnesium to be there when needed. That's a tall order for a nutrient that 68 percent of Americans fail to consume in sufficient quantities. In fact, according to the National Health and Nutrition Examination Survey (1999-2000), 19 percent of Americans do not consume even 50 percent of the recommended amount of this critical nutrient.

Many of magnesium's functions are associated with migraine and related symptoms. Let's look at a few of the main activities of this important mineral.

Magnesium and Calcium

Many times when you read or hear about taking magnesium supplements, calcium is usually mentioned as well. One reason for this association is that these two minerals have a special relationship that allows them to perform very important functions in the body, and it is critical that these substances maintain a healthy balance (calcium/magnesium ratio) to do their work. On a basic level, for example, calcium is needed for muscle contraction, while magnesium is required for muscle relaxation.

For example, magnesium is needed for secretion of the parathyroid hormone, which helps maintain calcium balance (homeostasis). If either calcium or magnesium levels are too high, secretion of this hormone is hindered and homeostasis is not achieved. Magnesium has another role in calcium homeostasis: it serves as the vehicle that transports calcium and potassium (more about this mineral below) into and out of cells. If there is a deficiency of magnesium (e.g., if you take high amounts of calcium daily, as some women do because they are concerned about getting osteoporosis), an imbalance can develop between magnesium and calcium, which in turn can change the electrical status of the cell membranes, disrupt the transport of calcium and potassium, and cause an increase in the flow of calcium from outside the cells (extracellular) to inside the cells (intracellular space). The result is calcium overload, or calcium dominance. Conventional medicine tries to "fix" this excess situation by prescribing drugs called calcium channel blockers, which I discussed in chapter 3. Calcium dominance can be resolved naturally, however, by supplementing with magnesium to restore balance to the calcium/magnesium ratio.

Calcium dominance is common among people who are older than 35. Calcium can cause hyperexcitability of cell membranes, decrease their electrical stability, and decrease pain threshold—all actions that can contribute to migraine and which can be balanced by the restoration of magnesium. A dominance of calcium (which stimulates the sympathetic nervous system) is also characterized by insomnia, constipation, high blood pressure, and arrhythmia. All four of these symptoms, but especially the first two, are indications of an imbalance between the sympathetic and parasympathetic nervous systems and are found among migraineurs. Once we rebalance hormones and restore the proper activity of the sympathetic and parasympathetic nervous system, these conditions typically resolve or greatly improve.

Individuals, and especially women, often ask whether they can take calcium supplements while participating in the Migraine Cure. I do not recommend calcium until individuals have been migraine-free for at least three months. You should discuss the appropriate dose with your physician and always take it with a balanced amount of magnesium. Additional magnesium should be taken at bedtime to stimulate the parasympathetic system.

Magnesium and Potassium

Magnesium and potassium also have a close relationship that can impact migraine. You need a healthy level of magnesium for the proper function of the sodium/potassium pump, a process whereby magnesium helps pump sodium out of cells and pump potassium into cells. Magnesium supplementation can normalize the levels of magnesium and potassium in the muscle cells. In a 2005 study at McGill University in Montreal, researchers noted that the sodium pump maintains a level of potassium that is critical for the propagation of electrical signals along nerve cells, and also found that reduced efficiency of the sodium/potassium pump is linked with migraine.

The Calcium/Magnesium Ratio

The relationship between the calcium/magnesium ratio and migraine has been known for some time. In 1993, for example, Mauskop and his colleagues published an article in Headache in which they noted that low levels of ionized magnesium and high ionized calcium/ionized magnesium ratio are both associated with migraine, as these two conditions cause cerebral vasospasm and reduced blood flow to the brain. In 1998, Mauskop again looked at the relationship between magnesium and migraine in a review of a large number of clinical and experimental studies and stated that "the importance of magnesium in the pathogenesis of migraine headaches is clearly established" and that "magnesium concentration has an effect on serotonin receptors . . . and a variety of other migraine related receptors and neurotransmitters." He also stated that lowered levels of ionized magnesium are present in up to half of patients during an acute migraine attack.

More recently, Dr. Mauskop explored the calcium/magnesium relationship in 341 women with migraine or headache. What he found lead him to state that the high incidence of ionized magnesium deficiency and elevated calcium/magnesium ratio seen during menstrual migraine confirm that a magnesium deficiency has a role in the development of menstrual migraine.

A balanced ration of calcium to magnesium also is necessary to help prevent fatigue (which it does by normalizing mitochondrial oxidation) and to regulate the sleep cycle, two factors common among migraineurs. Again, this balance also reflects a balance between the sympathetic nervous system (which calcium has an impact on) and the parasympathetic nervous system (which magnesium influences).

Steroid Hormones, Magnesium, and Calcium

Steroid hormones have an impact on the metabolism of magnesium and calcium. Estrogens, for example, regulate calcium metabolism, absorption of calcium in the intestinal tract, and increase parathyroid hormone gene expression and parathyroid hormone secretion, all of which have an effect on the menstrual cycle. Both estrogen and progesterone can have a significant impact on magnesium levels, although testosterone does not.

The relationships work the other way as well. When there is an imbalance between calcium and magnesium, the polarity of the cell membranes changes. This in turn disrupts the electrical stability of the cell membranes that I mentioned earlier, and their sensitivity to signals from the steroid hormones. When that happens, communication breaks down among the hormones and these two minerals, and an imbalance occurs.

Magnesium and Energy Production

Magnesium has a key role in the production of energy. Studies show that 93 percent of migraineurs also have chronic fatigue syndrome, therefore it is clear that magnesium can have a significant impact on improving energy levels. Indeed, nearly every individual who participates in the Migraine Cure reports significant improvements in energy and vitality after as little as a week of treatment.

A dramatic increase in energy was "the second best thing the Migraine Cure did for me," says Allison, a thirty-nine-year-old bookkeeper from Seattle. "Naturally, getting rid of my migraines was number one. But I can't believe how much energy I have now. I'm told the magnesium supplement is a big reason, and all I can say is, this stuff is great!"

Magnesium's impact on energy is due to its work inside cells in organelles ("little organs") called mitochondria, where magnesium helps cells manufacture ATP (adenosine triphosphate), the molecules that contain energy. Magnesium binds to these molecules, and once ATP is produced, magnesium then helps break it down so the energy can be released. The relationship between magnesium and ATP is critical, because without ATP, nutrients and other substances would not be able to move in and out of cells, metabolism would cease, and no energy would be produced.

Magnesium, the Nervous System, and Stress

Magnesium is critical for regulation of the central nervous system. In chapter 1, I explained that neuron hyperexcitability is one theory for a cause of migraine. In fact, research shows that low levels of magnesium in the brain can be an indication of a hyperactive, or excitable, nervous system and is associated with a greater risk for migraine. If you experience shakiness or tremors, if you get irritable or restless during the day, or if you wake up often during the night, these are all indications of low magnesium levels. This is one reason why you should take your magnesium supplement before going to bed.

During times of stress, levels of the stress hormone cortisol increase while magnesium levels decline, and levels of both magnesium and potassium in urine increase. Studies show that magnesium supplementation can reduce cortisol as well as adrenaline levels, which in turn helps control stress and its damaging effects.

Magnesium is also important (along with vitamin B6) in the production of serotonin, which not only is a critical mood-enhancing chemical, but is also a precursor of melatonin (see chapter 5).

Magnesium and the Heart

The health of the heart and the cardiovascular system depend a great deal on maintaining a proper magnesium level in the body. Magnesium helps coordinate heart muscle activity and the functioning of the nerves that initiate the heart beat. Overall, magnesium has a relaxing effect on blood vessels and smooth muscle (which includes heart muscle) and helps prevent spasm of the coronary arteries, a condition known as angina pectoris. It has a beneficial effect on blood pressure because it helps equalize the levels of sodium and potassium in the blood. Because magnesium helps deliver oxygen to working muscles, it has a role in protecting against myocardial infarction, cardiac arrhythmia, high blood pressure, and ischemic heart disease.

The components of the Migraine Cure are also key in reducing or eliminating risk factors for coronary heart disease in women. I discuss this approach in chapter 9.

Magnesium and Other Nutrients

Magnesium activates some of the B vitamins, especially B1 (thiamine) and B6, and is essential for the proper absorption of B6. If you'll recall, vitamin B6 is one of the nutrients that we recommend as a supplement, along with melatonin, as part of the Migraine Cure. It is important to maintain healthy levels of both vitamins B1 and B6, as deficiencies of these nutrients cause a reduction in the absorption of magnesium. Magnesium also has a part in the synthesis of protein.

How the Body Uses Magnesium

Approximately one-third to one-half of the magnesium you get in your diet and/or through supplements is absorbed in the small intestines and then transported through the bloodstream to cells in tissues and organs. Thus you want to maintain a healthy gut to help ensure proper absorption and ultimately the best utilization of magnesium. Gastrointestinal disorders such as Crohn's disease, irritable bowel syndrome, colitis, and chronic diarrhea and/or vomiting can result in magnesium deficiency.

Other factors that have a negative impact on the body's ability to absorb magnesium include high intake of protein, fat, sugar, and phosphates; alcohol consumption; and a deficiency of vitamins B1 and B6. Use of oral contraceptives and caffeine consumption increase the amount of magnesium you excrete in urine, while a diet that consists of a lot of processed and refined products helps ensure you won't get enough magnesium from your food. Although healthy kidneys can help compensate for poor dietary intake of magnesium by limiting the amount of magnesium that is excreted, they cannot stem the excessive loss of the mineral when such loss is related to the use of some medications or in people who have poorly controlled diabetes or alcoholism.

If a magnesium deficiency is part of the recipe for migraine, then it follows that supplementation should be beneficial, and research and experience indicate that this is true. Several studies have shown that supplementation with magnesium relieves migraine in people who have low serum ionized magnesium levels. We also know that supplementation with magnesium relieves symptoms of PMS, including migraine, bloating, and edema and that magnesium supplementation can be an effective prophylactic (preventive agent) and treatment for migraine.

Restoring the Magnesium/Calcium Ratio

Although magnesium supplements are available in a variety of types and forms (e.g., magnesium sulfate, oxide, gluconate, carbonate, chloride) the form of magnesium I recommend to everyone who participates in the Migraine Cure is magnesium citrate. This is the type the body is best able to absorb. Magnesium oxide is usually the least expensive type, but it also is the most poorly absorbed. I especially recommend a powdered, water-soluble magnesium supplement, 400 to 800 mg taken at bedtime, or 200 to 400 mg taken in the morning followed by 400 mg at bedtime, depending on the individual's needs. Magnesium is more available to the body when it is taken in water than it is in the diet, which is why I recommend a water-soluble form. Some people experience diarrhea when taking magnesium, but this symptom typically resolves if you reduce the dose. If you have any type of heart or kidney disease, talk to your doctor before taking magnesium.

Some patients ask which foods are rich sources of magnesium and whether they should include these in their diet. Magnesium-rich foods should always be a part of a balanced diet. Some excellent sources include almonds, cashews, soybeans, dark-green, leafy vegetables, halibut, baked potatoes, and peanuts. However, increasing your dietary intake of magnesium is not sufficient to restore low magnesium levels to normal. The magnesium supplement recommended as part of the Migraine Cure is, in my experience, the most effective in restoring balance to the calcium/magnesium ratio and, by extension, to the sympathetic/parasympathetic nervous systems.

In Conclusion

One simple mineral; how important can it be in the migraine program? What if you decide not to take it? The magnesium component, like the other components of the Migraine Cure, is a vital part of the entire plan. Remember the automobile analogy: leaving out the magnesium component is like inflating three out of four tires on your car. You still have a car, you can still drive it (albeit very slowly), but you need to inflate the fourth tire to make the car move properly.

When you supplement with magnesium citrate, you give your body one of the critical elements it needs to not only eliminate migraine, but contribute to your overall health and well-being.

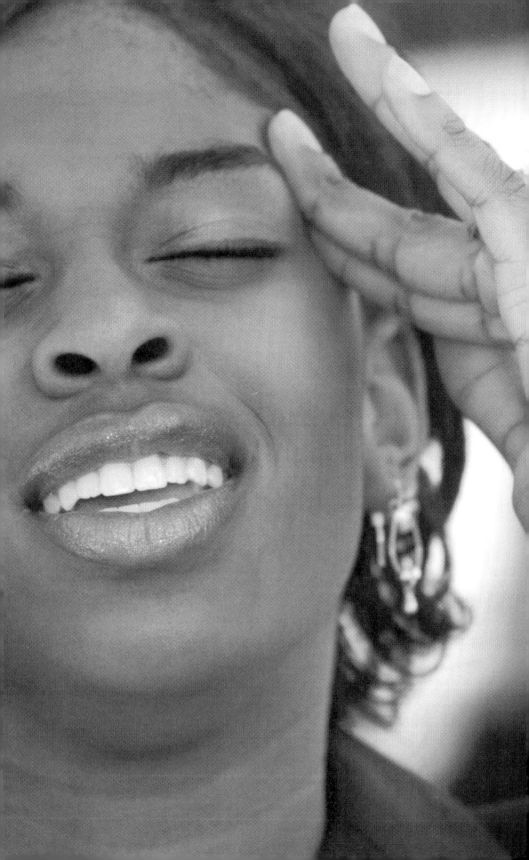

8

Three Stories

"This program saved my life and gave it back to me." This senti-
ment comes from Bettina, one of the former migraineurs whose
story appears in this chapter. She, along with many other men and women
who have participated in the Migraine Cure, have been very eager to talk
about the success they've had with the program and have expressed a desire
to tell their stories. Therefore in this chapter I share stories from three "vet-
eran" migraineurs: people who lived with the syndrome for a total of more
than 120 years before they found effective, lasting relief.

Bettina's Story

The migraines started around age eleven or twelve, recalls Bettina, as
she gazes out at the Atlantic Ocean from her waterfront home in Maine.
Now, for the first time in nearly a half century, she is virtually migraine-free
and nearly headache-free. "I feel like somebody gave me a new head," she
says.

When the headaches first started, Bettina says she refused to believe that
she might have migraines and kept telling herself that her head pain was
simply bad tension headaches. Her resistance stemmed from the fact that
she witnessed her mother's nearly daily struggle with migraines, and Bettina
didn't want to believe she might be slated for the same fate. As the years
passed, however, it became obvious that she, indeed, did have migraines.

Determined not to let them rule her life, however, Bettina went on to college, completed her degree in marine biology, got married, and went on to have a successful career.

By her mid-twenties, Bettina was having 12 to 18 migraines each month. Along with the head pain came constipation ("I was constipated my entire life") and gastrointestinal problems. After she underwent a partial hysterectomy at age 27, her doctor prescribed an estrogen patch. In the ensuing years, however, she began to experience vaginal dryness and a loss of sex drive, which were still complaints when she contacted us.

Throughout the years, Bettina had tried a wide variety of treatments, none of which offered any lasting relief. "Some things would work for a few days, and then I'd be right back where I was before," she says. "I went to an acupuncturist, a massage therapist, and a chiropractor. I tried herbs and vitamin pills. I tried beta-blockers, antidepressants, and calcium channel blockers. Nothing helped.

"In 1995 I tried sumatriptan [Imitrex®] injections, and the first time I gave myself an injection, I thought I had found the answer. I was nearly pain-free within minutes. But then eight or nine hours later I got a rebound migraine, and it was worse than the one I had stopped earlier. And because the pain was so bad I gave myself another injection and hoped that the rebound migraine was just a one-time occurrence. But it wasn't. Every time I used sumatriptan I got a rebound migraine within hours and I'd need another injection. I finally stopped using sumatriptan because it wasn't working and it was getting too expensive."

Discouraged by the lack of success with her latest treatment option, Bettina says "I became terrified—I saw no way out. I never had a good day." She began keeping a diary of the frequency of her migraines, some of which lasted more than 24 hours, and it reads like a horror story: 140 migraines in 1999; 91 in 2000; 98 in 2001; 124 in 2002; 108 in 2003; and 142 in 2004. It was in August 2004 that Bettina read an article I had written about migraine and the treatment program using hormone restoration. In that article I described migraine as a multisystem failure, and that was the defining moment for Bettina.

"That grabbed me," says Bettina. "Finally, a doctor who understood the concept, who had the big picture about migraine. I had to find out more." She contacted Life Extension that same day and poured out her story to one of our advisors. At that time she mentioned that a few months prior she had started herself on a program of DHEA (30 mg), pregnenolone (50 mg), and progesterone cream (dose unknown), along with the estrogen patch, which she had been using since her partial hysterectomy.

We were sure we could help Bettina and recommended she undergo lipid and hormone profiles, which she did immediately. Her results were as follows (reference ranges are in parentheses).

- Total cholesterol: 219 mg/dL (<200 mg/dL)
- Total estrogen: 286 pg/mL (61-437 pg/mL)
- Progesterone: 0.7 ng/mL (0.2-28 ng/mL)
- Total testosterone: 47 ng/dL (14-76 ng/dL)
- DHEA-S: 107 ug/dL (65-380 ug/dL)
- Pregnenolone: 125 ng/dL (10-230 ng/dL)

Based on the above report, we recommended the following program:

- Pregnenolone: 200 mg in the morning
- DHEA: 100 mg in the morning
- 7-Keto DHEA: 100 mg in the morning
- Probiotic formula, which contains 3.5 billion *Lactobacillus* group (*L. rhamnosus A, L. rhamnosus B, L. acidophilus, L. casei, L. bulgaricus*), 1.0 billion *Bifidobacterium* group (*B. longum, B. breve*), and 0.5 billion *Streptococcus thermophilus*, as well as gluten-free grasses, algae, natural fiber, herbs, and bioflavonoid extracts; one dose (1 scoop) in the morning
- Melatonin formula containing 3 mg of melatonin, 250 mg kava root extract, and 10 mg vitamin B6; two capsules before bedtime for one week, then one capsule at bedtime

- Magnesium citrate formula, one scoop (containing 420 mg) at bedtime
- Estrogens: Triest®, formulated to 90% estriol, 7% estradiol, and 3% estrone gel, used on a cyclical basis: 0.8 mL in the morning on days 1 through 14 of each month, then 0.6 mL in the morning on days 15 through 25, then 0.4 mL in the morning for the remainder of each month (five to six days)
- Micronized progesterone (50 mg/mL) gel used on a cyclical basis: 0.8 mL in the morning and 0.2 mL in the evening on days 1 through 14, then 1.0 mL in the morning and 0.2 mL in the evening on days 15 through 25, then 0.6 mL in the morning and 0.2 in the evening for the remainder of each month (five to six days)
- Micronized testosterone (50 mg/mL) gel, 0.2 mL in the morning for five days, then 0.1 mL every day
- Saw palmetto: 160 mg in the morning
- Zinc: 30 mg at bedtime

Eager to begin her treatment, Bettina gathered together the recommended supplements and tried to find a physician who would prescribe the bio-identical hormones. That's when she ran into a roadblock.

"I couldn't find a doctor who would prescribe the bio-identical estrogens I needed," she says. "My gynecologist refused and so did a few other doctors that I approached. They all said the synthetic hormones were fine. When I finally did find a doctor who was willing to write a prescription, it was for an estrogen-progesterone-testosterone combination gel that wasn't what had been recommended." By this time Bettina had spent nearly two months trying to get the right hormones, and she was getting frustrated. Although the formulation wasn't right, she began to use the three-hormone combination gel and hoped for some positive results.

After using the combination gel for one month and not experiencing any improvement, she stopped using it and purchased an over-the-counter progesterone gel (Pro Fem®), which she applied in the following manner: 1/2 teaspoon the first 1 to 14 days of the month, 1 teaspoon on days 15 through 25, and 1/3 teaspoon from day 26 until the end of the month. She contacted us near the end of her first month on this program and the other supplements we had recommended (except the estrogens and testosterone) and said that her migraines were less severe and less frequent, and that her digestion and sleep were somewhat improved.

Bettina still needed to find the right hormones, however, and so she continued her search for a cooperative physician. Finally, five months after she first contacted us, Bettina's persistence paid off, and she began the full program with the correct hormones. After only two weeks on the Migraine Cure, Bettina called us to say that for the first time in decades, she had been migraine-free for eight days. "I couldn't believe it," she says. "I finally felt like there was hope."

That was April 2005, and nearly one year later, Bettina says her life has completely turned around. "I have lots of energy, I can eat chocolate and caffeine. I have no sleep or digestive problems." And although she gets an occasional mild headache, she doesn't get migraines. She is still taking a modified version of the original recommendations, including 50 mg of DHEA, 50 mg of 7-Keto, 100 mg of pregnenolone, and the estrogens, progesterone, and testosterone. Her cholesterol, which she describes as "always being high" is less than 220 mg/dL.

"This program saved my life and gave it back to me," she says.

Ruthanne's Story

"I've had migraines as long as I can remember," says Ruthanne, a fifty-one-year-old self-employed graphic artist. She is sitting near the window of her home office, which offers her a spectacular view of the sky over the Texas panhandle. Until recently she watched that sky with trepidation, as her daily migraines were often triggered by changes in the weather.

Ruthanne first contacted us in October 2004, when she told her story. "The migraines actually started when I was about fifteen," she says, "and in the last ten years or so they got worse, until I was having one every day." She remembers that her teenage years were plagued by symptoms of premenstrual syndrome, including migraine, depression, and mood swings, and at nineteen she began to take birth control pills to help deal with the PMS. That's when she noticed that although she still got migraines when she was taking the pills, they were much worse during the one week per month that she was off the hormones. This trend continued for all the years Ruthanne took the birth control pills, which was up until the time she started the Migraine Cure.

Over the years, Ruthanne says she tried various medications to cope with the migraines, including naratriptan (Amerge®), which she sometimes needed twice a day and to which she built up a tolerance. She also tried sumatriptan (Imitrex®), topiramate (Topamax®, an anticonvulsant), various muscle relaxants, several different antidepressants, ergotamine injections, and a few different hormone replacement formulations, all of which provided little or no relief.

Despite the nearly daily migraines, Ruthanne continued to work at home and to participate in one of her few pleasures, swimming. At the time she contacted us, her other health concerns included allergies ("I've always been highly allergic to different foods, chemicals, and airborne particles"), high blood pressure (140/90), and overweight (215 pounds at 5'4").

As a result of Ruthanne's consultation with our advisors, it was recommended that she undergo blood tests to determine her lipid and hormone levels. Her results were as follows:

- Cholesterol: 296 mg/dL (<200 mg/dL)
- Total estrogen: 146 pg/mL (61 – 437 pg/mL)
- Progesterone: 0.3 ng/mL (0.2 – 28.0 ng/mL)
- Pregnenolone: 37 ng/dL (10 – 230 ng/dL)
- DHEA-S: 76 ug/dL (65 – 380 ug/dL)
- Total testosterone: 32 ng/dL (14 – 75 ng/dL)

Based on these results and the information we gathered during our discussion with Ruthanne, we recommended the following initial program:

- DHEA: 50 mg in the morning and 25 mg at noon
- 7-Keto DHEA: 100 mg in the morning
- Pregnenolone: 200 mg in the morning
- Estrogens: Triest gel, formulated to 90% estriol, 7% estradiol, and 3% estrone, taken on a cyclical basis: 1 mL in the morning on days 1 through 10 following menstruation, then 0.8 mL in the morning until start of menstruation, then 0.4 mL in the morning during menses
- Progesterone: micronized progesterone (50 mg/mL), 0.8 mL in the morning and 0.4 mL in the evening for days 1 through 10 following menstruation, then 1.0 mL in the morning and 0.4 mL in the evening until start of menstruation, then 0.6 mL in the morning and 0.2 mL in the evening during menses
- Testosterone: micronized testosterone (50 mg/mL) gel, 0.2 mL in the morning for days 1 through 10 following menstruation, then 0.1 mL every day
- Probiotic formula, which contains 3.5 billion *Lactobacillus* group (*L. rhamnosus A, L. rhamnosus B, L. acidophilus, L. casei, L. bul-*

garicus), 1.0 billion *Bifidobacterium* group (*B. longum*, *B. breve*), and 0.5 billion *Streptococcus thermophilus*, as well as gluten-free grasses, algae, natural fiber, herbs, and bioflavonoid extracts; one dose (1 scoop) in the morning
- Melatonin formula containing 3 mg of melatonin, 250 mg kava root extract, and 10 mg vitamin B6; one capsule at bedtime
- Magnesium citrate formula, one scoop (containing 420 mg) at bedtime
- Saw palmetto, 160 mg in the morning
- Zinc, 50 mg before bedtime

We also recommended that Ruthanne stop taking her supplements (including calcium and a multiple vitamin/mineral) and her birth control pills (she was still menstruating) until her hormone levels were restored. This request made her very anxious, as she was very afraid that once she stopped the birth control pills, her moods would be "out of control" and that she would experience feelings of detachment, a feeling she often had whenever she was not taking the pills. We tried to reassure her that once she started to take the hormones recommended in the program, her hormone levels would be restored and these feelings would not be an issue.

While Ruthanne wrestled with her anxiety about stopping her birth control pills, another issue came up: her gynecologist would not prescribe the bio-identical estrogens she needed. Thus began Ruthanne's one-year search for a physician who would prescribe the bio-identical hormones for her. (Note: This is not typical. Unfortunately, Ruthanne lives in an area in which any type of nonconventional, complementary medical care is hard to find. Many individuals who participate in the Migraine Cure have little or no trouble finding a health-care professional who will write a prescription for them. See "Resources" in the appendix for help finding a physician.) In the end, she found a nurse practitioner who was not only happy to provide the prescription, but who was also interested in the program, as she suffered with migraines as well.

Ruthanne remembers the exact day—November 19, 2005—that she started the Migraine Cure program. And for good reason. "From day 1, I didn't have any more migraines," she says. "It worked immediately. Although I still get some headaches, they go away with an aspirin. I can't remember when I was migraine-free like this!" She was also greatly relieved that her concerns about stopping the birth control pills had been unfounded: her mood was good and she continued to feel positive.

Ruthanne also had this to say about some other benefits of the program. "With all the medications I used to take just to get by, I was 'fuzzy' all the time, to the point that I believed that was my normal state. But now my mind is sharper, clearer, and I feel like I am right there in life again instead of feeling like an observer." She warns others that, like her, they may experience a worsening memory for a brief time before feeling better.

"For a month or so after I was off all the drugs I felt like my memory was getting worse, or I couldn't remember words," she says. "It was a little frightening." Then she learned that such memory problems are typical when someone transitions from a medicated to a nonmedicated state, and that her memory problems would be temporary. "Now, I feel sharper than I have for a long, long time, and I attribute it to not being on migraine drugs and pain killers and to finally getting my hormones into balance."

As of February 2006, Ruthanne had been migraine-free for three full months and reported having much more energy, improved sleep, a positive mood, no feelings of detachment, and a big improvement in her allergies. Her blood pressure was a healthy 112/84, and she was looking into incorporating more healthy foods into her diet.

Hillary's Story

When Hillary first contacted us in December 2004, you could literally hear the fatigue, despair, and pain in her voice through the phone. For thirty-eight of her fifty-six years, Hillary had experienced migraines; at first, one or two a month, then gradually increasing until they were occurring daily. Like many migraineurs, she chose not to use prescription medications for the pain and associated symptoms and instead attempted to manage them with various over-the-counter pain killers. The only time Hillary had been nearly migraine-free was when she was pregnant: she had had two normal pregnancies and five abortions.

Along with the head pain Hillary said she also had long suffered with depression, sleep disturbances, muscle aches, hypertension, chronic fatigue, severe hot flashes, and lack of sex drive. She was overweight (187 pounds and 5'2") and said that her most significant weight gain—more than 20 pounds—had occurred when she was around thirty-five, at the same time she began to experience symptoms of premenstrual syndrome. Her menstrual cycle stopped at age fifty-two.

Around the time her menses stopped, Hillary was diagnosed with high blood pressure (150/95 mmHg) and extremely high cholesterol (greater than 300 mg/dL). Her doctor prescribed nadolol for her blood pressure and a statin drug (atorvastatin; Lipitor) for her high cholesterol. The atorvastatin "made me feel even worse than I already felt," said Hillary. "My stomach was always upset, and I was also worried about liver damage, so I quit taking the drug after two months." She did, however, continue with the nadolol.

Hillary was told about our migraine program through a friend, and she called us the very same day. After what she called a "very long, very thorough telephone conversation" with one of our health advisors, Hillary arranged for blood testing through her primary care physician and had the results sent to us. Her results were as follows (reference ranges are in parentheses):

- Total cholesterol: 300 mg/dL (<200 mg/dL)
- Estradiol: 19 pg/mL (19-528 pg/mL)
- Progesterone: 0.4 ng/mL (0.2 – 28.0 ng/mL)
- Total testosterone: 51 ng/dL (14-75 ng/dL)
- DHEA-S: 86 ug/dL (65-380 ng/dL)
- Pregnenolone: <10 ng/dL (10-230 ng/dL)

Based on the information Hillary gave us and her test results, we recommended the following initial program:

- Pregnenolone, 200 mg in the morning
- DHEA, 50 mg in the morning
- 7-Keto DHEA, 100 mg in the morning
- Saw palmetto, 160 mg in the morning
- Zinc, 30 mg at bedtime
- Probiotic formula, which contains 3.5 billion *Lactobacillus* group (*L. rhamnosus A, L. rhamnosus B, L. acidophilus, L. casei, L. bulgaricus*), 1.0 billion *Bifidobacterium* group (*B. longum, B. breve*), and 0.5 billion *Streptococcus thermophilus*, as well as gluten-free grasses, algae, natural fiber, herbs, and bioflavonoid extracts; one dose (1 scoop) in the morning
- Melatonin formula containing 3 mg of melatonin, 250 mg kava root extract, and 10 mg vitamin B6; one capsule at bedtime
- Magnesium citrate formula, one scoop (containing 420 mg) at bedtime
- Estrogens: Triest gel, formulated to 90% estriol, 7% estradiol, and 3% estrone, taken on a cyclical basis: 1.0 mL in the morning on days 1 through 14 of each month, then 0.8 mL in the morning on days 15 through 25, then 0.6 mL in the morning for the remaining five to six days of each month
- Progesterone: Micronized progesterone (50 mg/mL) gel used on a cyclical basis: 0.8 mL in the morning and 0.4 mL in the evening for days 1 through 14 of each month, then 1.0 mL in the morning and 0.4 mL in the evening for days 15 through 25 of each month, then 0.6 mL in the morning and 0.2 mL in the evening for the remaining five to six days of each month

We asked Hillary to contact us again in four weeks to let us know how she was feeling so we could make any necessary adjustments to her program. Weeks four and five came and went, and Hillary had not yet called. When she finally contacted us six weeks after starting the program, she apologized, saying "I'm feeling so great and I've been so excited that I just got caught up in doing things I've been wanting to do for such a long time!" At the top of her list for why she felt "great" was the fact that she was migraine-free for the first time in thirty-eight years. She also said she had stopped taking all her pain medication, her energy level was significantly better, and her sex drive had returned.

We suggested that Hillary have her lipid and hormone levels checked again in about three to four months and asked her to let us know how she was doing with the program so we could make any adjustments. She contacted us in October 2005, ten months after starting the program, and said that her total cholesterol was an impressive 195 mg/dL. "My doctor can't believe it," she said. "I did it without drugs!" She was still migraine-free and said that all her other symptoms were either completely or nearly gone. "Now that I'm pain-free and I have the energy to exercise, I'm losing weight," she said. "I feel like a completely new person."

In Conclusion

Three women, each with a long history of migraine, and each with a different—but similar—migraine program. One interesting thing about the Migraine Cure is that although there are very specific components that must be included in the program for it to be effective, there is also much flexibility in the doses and in the length of time any one dose or supplement is given. I like to say that the treatment evolves as balance resolves. Each of the former migraineurs in this chapter is now on a maintenance program that differs from the program that was first recommended. Thus, the Migraine Cure program is adjusted to meet the unique needs of each individual.

What will your program look like? To find out, you need to contact us, get hormone and lipid profiles, and share the results with us. Together we can eliminate migraine.

9

Additional Uses And Benefits Of The Migraine Cure Program

Expect the unexpected. When you're talking about the Migraine Cure, the unexpected comes in the form of bonus health benefits. One of the most rewarding things about the Migraine Cure, besides the fact that it eliminates migraine, is that it also alleviates so many other symptoms and conditions. This is good news, because most people who live with migraine also struggle with one or more other health problems, including depression, insomnia, high cholesterol, constipation, irritable bowel syndrome, chronic fatigue, fibromyalgia, mood swings, menstrual difficulties, or sleep disturbances. So while we were busy recommending hormone restoration, pineal resetting, calcium/magnesium rebalancing, and digestive realignment and getting excellent results when it came to eliminating migraine, patients were reporting—and we were noting—that other health concerns were disappearing as well.

"It was goodbye migraine, and goodbye fatigue, crankiness, and depression," says Madison, a twenty-eight-year-old lab technician who had suffered with migraines since age 15. "I thought, 'wow, the migraines are gone AND all these other symptoms disappear too.' That's more than I expected."

"Irritable bowel was such a constant problem, along with the migraine, that I didn't' even separate the two," says Stephanie, a thirty-seven-year-old mother of two. "So when the migraines stopped, I said to myself, 'hey, my gut is feeling better, too. Is that possible? ' And according to Dr. Dzugan, yes! I feel like I got a bonus!"

Forty-year-old Pamela says her entire life has changed. "I had migraine and fibromyalgia for years, my cholesterol was way too high, and I was overweight" she says. "I had to quit my job, and I stayed home a lot. My kids suffered, my husband suffered, and I just wanted to die. Now the migraines and fibromyalgia are gone, my cholesterol is within normal range, and I've lost a few pounds. I've gone back to work and I've taken up tennis. I used to think my life was over, but boy, was I wrong. Life is good!"

My research and experience have shown me that the basics of the Migraine Cure—hormone restoration, pineal gland resetting, digestive system modification, and calcium/magnesium rebalancing—are the recipe for successful treatment and often complete elimination of many other physical and psychological conditions. In this chapter I share with you some of that research and, more importantly, what the findings can mean to you and your loved ones who may be living with high cholesterol, heart disease, or fibromyalgia.

High Cholesterol

High cholesterol, or hypercholesterolemia, is defined as a total cholesterol level of 200 mg/dL (milligrams of cholesterol per deciliter of blood) or greater. A desirable range is 160 to 199 mg/dL.

Hypercholesterolemia can cause the development and accumulation of plaque—cholesterol, other fatty substances, calcium, and fibrous tissue—in the arteries, which blocks the flow of blood and can result in coronary heart disease or atherosclerosis, which can lead to pieces of plaque breaking away from the artery walls and increasing the risk for stroke, heart attack, circulation problems, and death.

Hypercholesterolemia and Migraine

I have seen it again and again: when people with migraine also have high cholesterol (and the majority of them do), and they follow the recommendations outlined in the Migraine Cure, their cholesterol levels normalize. Let me give you an example.

Between 1999 and 2005, Arnold R. Smith, MD, and I treated and followed up on 30 patients who had migraine. The patients ranged in age from 16 to 66 years, and they had had migraine for a range of 2 to 46 years. When the individuals underwent the hormone and lipid panels at the beginning of the study, we found that 27 of them had abnormal cholesterol levels: 24 (80%) had high cholesterol (hypercholesterolemia), and 3 had low cholesterol (hypocholesterolemia; levels below 160 mg/dL are associated with poor production of steroid hormones).

All the patients followed the program as I have outlined in previous chapters: bio-identical hormone restoration accompanied by supplementation with melatonin, kava root extract, vitamin B6, magnesium, and a probiotic formula, each according to his or her personal needs. Not only did all of the patients become migraine-free, but 22 of the 24 patients who had had high cholesterol at the beginning of the study achieved normal cholesterol levels.

We had similar findings in another study, published in *Medical Hypotheses* in 2002. In that study we reported on twenty patients with hypercholesterolemia (mean total cholesterol, 263.5 mg/dL) who also had suboptimal levels of steroidal hormones. All of the patients were given hormone restorative therapy, and all twenty responded well to treatment. In fact, 60 percent of them achieved a total cholesterol level of less than 200 mg/dL.

Michael's Story

One of the most interesting and challenging cases of hypercholesterolemia that responded to hormone restoration involved Michael, a thirty-four-year-old exporter who, along with his wife, contacted me and said he had an inherited form of extremely high cholesterol, and could I help him. Michael explained that his father, who was in his seventies, also had this condition, but that he refused to retire from running the chain of clothing stores he had in New York City. Michael and his wife were concerned, however, that perhaps Michael wouldn't be so lucky and that a heart attack could be on the horizon.

"I've heard so many terrible things about statin drugs," said Michael's wife, Peggy, "that we don't want to resort to using them. But Michael has been eating a fat-free diet with no red meat and no eggs for many years. He exercises regularly. Still the cholesterol is sky high [greater than 500 mg/dL]. His ophthalmologist checked his eyes and told him the blood vessels in the back of his eyes look like they belong to someone in their sixties! We need to do something, but we don't know what it is."

I told Michael and Peggy that based on my clinical experience, Michael's problem was not familial hypercholesterolemia, but rather familial low hormone production. This caught their attention. We then discussed hormone restoration therapy, and Michael was skeptical but agreed to try it. For the next three months, Michael took 50 mg DHEA, 100 mg pregnenolone (both to address the suboptimal levels seen on his hormone profile results), a multivitamin, and 100 mg coenzymeQ10 (the latter because of its effectiveness in the prevention and treatment of heart disease). At the end of three months, Michael's cholesterol level had dropped to 350. Michael and Peggy were hopeful, and I suggested increasing the DHEA to 100 mg and the pregnenolone to 200 mg.

Three months passed, and when Michael had his cholesterol checked again, it had risen to 400, and Michael admitted he had not been taking his supplements regularly. Peggy became upset, and Michael agreed to recommit to the treatment program. At this point I recommended increasing pregnenolone to 300 mg, and also adding 600 mg of N-acetylcysteine (NAC), a form of the amino acid cysteine and an antioxidant that is helpful in the support and enhancement of liver function. I added the NAC because of the results of some previous laboratory results. It seems that in the past, whenever Michael had taken niacin to help lower his cholesterol, his liver enzymes would rise, and he would have to stop taking the niacin. This information lead me to believe that Michael's familial hypercholesterolemia was actually a genetic defect that was showing up as a dysfunction of his liver — the main organ involved in internal production of cholesterol. It was worth a try.

Three months later, Michael's total cholesterol was 210 mg/dL—a remarkable figure for him — and his DHEA and pregnenolone were at suboptimal levels. Both Michael and Peggy are thrilled with the results, and Michael has promised to keep a close eye on his cholesterol. Blood tests showed that Michael's testosterone was very low (274 ng/dL; optimal 241 – 827 ng/dL), but he had not yet agreed to add this hormone to his program. We fully expect Michael's total cholesterol level to fall below 200 mg/dL once all the deficient hormones have been restored.

Coronary Heart Disease

Coronary heart disease (CHD) is the leading cause of death among women in the United States, a fact that still does not resonate with many women, and even some physicians. According to the American Heart Association, CHD causes the death of more than 241,000 women each year, about five times more deaths than those associated with breast cancer. For many, the idea that CHD is primarily a man's disease still persists. Yet there is another serious statistic well worth mentioning: the warning signs of CHD among women differ somewhat from those among men. Thus not only is women's risk of CHD failing to get the attention it deserves, women and health-care practitioners may be overlooking the warning signs.

WARNING SIGNS OF CHD

Generally, there are two types of risk factors for coronary heart disease: nonmodifiable and modifiable. Those in the first category include:

- Age: More than 83 percent of people who die of CHD are 65 years or older.
- Gender: Men are at greater risk of heart attack than women, and they have their attacks earlier in life. However, 38% of American women compared with 25% of American men die within one year of suffering a heart attack.
- Ethnicity: The risk of heart disease is greater among Mexican Americans, Native Americans, native Hawaiians, and some Asian Americans. African Americans have more severe high

blood pressure than Caucasians and thus a greater risk of heart disease.
- Family history: People with a family history (close relatives) of heart disease are more likely to develop the disease.

Risk factors in the modifiable category include the following:
- High cholesterol.
- High homocysteine (an amino acid that is associated with coronary heart disease, atherosclerosis, and stroke when present at high levels).
- High blood pressure.
- Diabetes.
- High C-reactive protein (CRP) (a protein that increases in the presence of systemic inflammation, thus testing CRP levels in the blood can help evaluate cardiovascular disease risk).
- Obesity or being overweight.
- Smoking.
- Sedentary lifestyle.
- High stress.
- Metabolic syndrome (a syndrome characterized by a combination of hypertension, insulin resistance, obesity, elevated C-reactive protein, and lipid disorder).

Compared with men, women tend to develop CHD later in life (after menopause), and it is believed that natural hormones (not synthetic hormone replacement therapy) may help protect women from CHD. Diabetes also increases a woman's risk of CHD three to seven times, compared with a two to three time greater risk among men.

The good news about coronary heart disease risk factors is that there are more you can change than not change. With that in mind, let's look at Karla's story and see how a version of the Migraine Cure was able to help her reduce her risk of coronary heart disease.

Karla's Story

At age fifty-three, Karla had a beautiful home in the suburbs, two bright and very successful sons, and a wide circle of friends. She also had a health profile that placed her on a collision course with disaster. The year was 2000.

That's the time Karla decided she had to look beyond conventional medicine for help with the long list of medical problems that had been plaguing her for more than a decade. Her health during her twenties and thirties had mostly been good, with the exception of a complete hysterectomy she had at age thirty because of severe fibroids. In the decade after the surgery, her health seemed to be satisfactory until she neared forty.

"That was my turning point year," she says. "I got a divorce, I was under a lot of stress, and everything healthwise seemed to start going wrong." Karla began experiencing various problems, including chronic fatigue, hypertension, depression, anxiety, panic attacks, insomnia, arthritis, hot flashes, loss of sex drive, vaginal yeast infections, muscle pain, severe shortness of breath, and short-term memory problems. Her weight, which had hovered around 115 pounds for many years, shot up to more than 200, which placed her in the "obese" category at her height of 5 feet. Her doctor diagnosed her with type II diabetes. Karla had the ingredients for a heart attack, and she knew it.

During Karla's initial interview, she told us she was taking two oral diabetes drugs, two antihypertension medications, bupropion (Wellbutrin®) for depression, Premarin® (synthetic hormone replacement) for hot flashes and loss of libido, acetaminophen for muscle pain, several weight-loss supplements, and several vitamin supplements. Our primary concern was that Karla was at high risk for coronary heart disease, and we explained that we could significantly reduce her risk by restoring selected hormone levels and restoring balance to her sympathetic and parasympathetic nervous systems. Therefore, we recommended she undergo a hormone panel, and the results were as follows:

- Total estrogen: 699 pg/mL (61-437 pg/mL)
- Progesterone: 0.2 ng/mL (0.2-28 ng/mL)
- Testosterone: 16 ng/dL (14-76 ng/dL)
- DHEA-S: 35 ug/dL (65-380 ug/dL)
- Pregnenolone: <10 ng/dL (10-230 ng/dL)

Karla was clearly in estrogen dominance, with an estrogen level that soared above the high end of the reference range and a progesterone level at the bottom. We immediately suggested she start with the following supplement plan, with all dosing taking place in the morning unless noted otherwise:

- Pregnenolone: 200 mg taken in the morning
- DHEA: 100 mg taken in the morning
- Estrogen: Triest gel, 1 mL on days 1 through 14 of each month, then 0.8 mL on days 15 through 25 of each month, then 0.4 mL on the last five to six days of each month
- Progesterone: micronized gel (50 mg/mL) taken as 0.8 mL on days 1 to 14 of each month; then 1.0 mL on days 15 to 25 of each month; and 0.6 mL on the last five to six days of each month
- Testosterone: micronized gel (50 mg/mL) taken as 0.2 mL every day
- Melatonin formula containing 3 mg of melatonin, 250 mg kava root extract, and 10 mg vitamin B6; one capsule at bedtime
- Vitamin E (1,000 IU) and selenium (200 mcg), both recommended for heart health
- Chromium: 400 mcg twice daily, to help with diabetes and weight loss

To help with weight loss, we also suggested she decrease the amount of carbohydrates in her diet and talk to her primary care physician about starting a regular exercise program.

Karla contacted us within a few days of starting the treatment program and said she had stopped taking the Premarin. When she called again four weeks later, it was hard for her to contain her enthusiasm. "I can't believe how good I feel," she said. "I feel ten years younger; I have energy, and I lost ten pounds. For so long I felt like my life was over, but now I'm hopeful." So hopeful, in fact, that she told her primary care doctor she was stopping her antidepressant. She had already stopped taking the acetaminophen, which she was anxious to do because she was afraid of possible liver damage from long-term use.

To help Karla feel even better, we recommended she add a few more supplements to her program:

- Glucosamine sulfate (2,250 mg taken daily in the morning) to help rebuild cartilage and relieve arthritis pain
- Additional progesterone (0.2 ml) one hour before bedtime. Progesterone helps stimulate the parasympathetic nervous system and thus aids sleep
- Magnesium citrate (420 mg) one hour before bedtime. Magnesium improves sleep and benefits the heart, and also helps restore balance to the magnesium/calcium ratio (see chapter 7)

Karla contacted us again four months later, and she had much good news to report. "Whenever I think, 'I don't want to exercise today' or 'gee, I have to take another supplement,' I just remember how great I feel, and that ends all my griping," she said. "The truth is, I feel like a different person than I was six months ago. My blood pressure is normal, something that hasn't happened in more than twelve years, even with medication. I lost an additional 28 pounds, and so for the first time in more than a decade I weigh less than 200 pounds. I'm well on my way to a healthier, slimmer me!"

To further encourage and support Karla's weight loss and exercise, we recommended she add the following supplements (all have been found to help reduce body fat and/or otherwise assist in weight loss) to her program until she reached her target weight of 140 pounds:

- Conjugated linoleic acid (CLA), 8 grams before breakfast
- Chitosan, two capsules before lunch and two before dinner
- Hydroxycitric acid (HCA), one 1,000-mg capsule three times daily before meals

We also suggested she add a B-complex vitamin, 3,000 mg of omega-3 fatty acids (taken twice daily), and that she use a one-month parasite-cleansing program. We sometimes recommend this cleansing program for individuals who continue to feel fatigued after being on the treatment program for several months. Parasites, which are present in the majority of Americans, are often a cause of fatigue and respond well to a mild, one-month cleansing treatment. In Karla's case, we wanted her to continue feeling good, and we did not want any lingering fatigue to dissuade her from pursuing her exercise program.

At her one-year follow-up visit, Karla was within twenty pounds of her target weight, she had stopped her diabetes medications, which meant she was now completely medication-free, and both her blood pressure and blood sugar levels were normal and stable. She also reported that she was dating again and "feeling very good about myself."

Fibromyalgia

Fibromyalgia is a condition characterized primarily by generalized joint and muscle pain that is not associated with any physical abnormality, tenderness in specific areas of the body, and fatigue. According to the American College of Rheumatology, a diagnosis of fibromyalgia should meet certain criteria; namely, that the soft tissue pain should be present for at least three months, and the individual should experience pain when pressure is applied to at least 11 of 18 specific sites, referred to as tender points, on the body. Other features often include sleep disturbances, depression, allergies, migraine, irritable bowel syndrome, memory problems, and sensitivity to stress and noise.

The cause of fibromyalgia is uncertain, but many theories have been put forth. Among them are those that point to a role by the hypothalamic-pituitary-adrenal (HPA) axis (see chapter 2), as well as a disturbance in hormone levels, both of which seem highly likely. Indeed, I propose that fibromyalgia is a result of an imbalance in neurohormones and metabolism and that hormone restoration and metabolic support may be key factors in regaining that balance.

Connie's Story

"It all started in the early 1980s with back pain that affected my upper spine right below my neck, and then my lower back," says Connie, a fifty-five-year-old former retail manager living in Tallahassee, Florida. "From then on, my life fell apart." Within a few months of the beginning of the back pain, Connie developed severe fatigue, migraine, persistent constipation, joint stiffness, poor short-term memory, insomnia, and panic attacks. At five-foot-six, her once trim 130-pound figure soon mushroomed to near 170. She noticed that her once very regular menstrual cycle had become highly irregular, and by the late 1980s her periods stopped completely, and so had her sex drive. Exhaustion, pain, and fear became a part of her daily life.

Connie sought help from several specialists, all of whom told her that there was nothing physically wrong with her and that her pain was "all in her head." Their answer to all her symptoms was for her to take medications, and plenty of them. Connie didn't want to rely solely on the drugs, so throughout the 1980s and 1990s she tried several different therapies, including acupuncture, chiropractic, massage, physical therapy, and exercise programs at various times, but none of them provided her with much improvement. It wasn't until 2000 that Connie finally received a diagnosis—fibromyalgia—from a rheumatologist. Connie described the diagnosis as a mixed blessing. "I was glad that someone finally believed that my pain wasn't just in my head," said Connie. "I felt 'validated,' and that was important. But at the same time I was extremely upset, because I realized I had already tried so many different drugs and therapies that are typically recommended for fibromyalgia, and none of them had worked."

Although she had felt depressed for years, the diagnosis plunged her into despair. One weekend in late 2000 she decided she had had enough, and she attempted suicide by taking an overdose of medications. Fortunately her family got her to the hospital in time, and before she left the hospital her doctor prescribed several antidepressants and a sleep aid.

By the time Connie came to us looking for help, she was taking several different pain killers, both prescription and over-the-counter, as well as bupropion (Wellbutrin®, an antidepressant), clonazepam (Klonopin®, an anticonvulsant also used for depression), zoldipem (Ambien®, a sleeping agent), and hormone replacement therapy containing estradiol and norethindrone acetate (Activella®). "I tried to keep working as long as I could," she said, "but often I felt like I was right on the edge, that I wouldn't be able to make it through another day. The drugs seemed to be the only things that made it possible for me to function." Eventually, however, she had quit her job, and at the time she came to see us she was working part-time in the office of her husband's general contracting business, "whenever I feel up to it."

After talking at length with Connie and documenting her personal and family medical histories (she had no family history of either fibromyalgia or migraine), we believed her symptoms were related to serious hormonal imbalance. We suggested she undergo blood tests to determine her hormone levels, with the following results (reference ranges in parentheses):

- DHEA-S: 100 ug/dL (65-380 ug/dL)
- Pregnenolone: 32 ng/dL (10-230 ng/dL)
- Total estrogen: 59 pg/mL (61-437 pg/mL)
- Progesterone: 0.6 ng/mL (0.2-28 ng/mL)
- Total testosterone: 50 ng/dL (14-76 ng/dL)

Based on these results, we recommended the following initial plan:
- Pregnenolone: 300 mg taken in the morning
- DHEA: 100 mg taken in the morning
- 7-keto DHEA: 70 mg taken at noon

- Estrogens: Triest® gel, which we recommended at a ratio of 90 percent estriol, 7 percent estradiol, and 3 percent estrone. The suggested dose, all to be taken in the morning, was 1 mL on days 1 through 14, 0.8 mL on days 15 through 25, and 0.4 mL on the remaining days of each month
- Progesterone(micronized) gel (50 mg/mL): The suggested dose, to be taken in the morning, was 0.8 mL on days 1 through 14 of each month, then 1.0 mL on days 15 through 25, then 0.6 mL on the remaining days of each month
- Testosterone gel (50 mg/mL): 0.2 mL in the morning every other day
- Melatonin mixture: two capsules, each containing 3 mg of melatonin, 250 mg of kava root extract, and 10 mg of vitamin B6, taken at bedtime
- Vitamin C-Magnesium supplement: two tablets containing a total of 1,860 mg of vitamin C, 100 mg of calcium, 40 mg of magnesium, 10 mg of vitamin B6, 72 mg of magnesium citrate, and 200 mg of bioflavonoids, taken at bedtime
- Glucosamine sulfate: 2,250 mg taken in the morning, for aches and pains
- A natural rheumatoid blend containing 10 mg undenatured type II collagen plus devil's claw root extract and bromelain, one capsule taken at bedtime (NOTE: Douglas laboratories Rheuma Shield™)

Within a week of beginning treatment, Connie stopped taking her hormone replacement therapy. At her one-month follow-up visit, Connie said her migraines were less frequent and severe, she was less fatigued, her depression had improved, and her back and joint pain were significantly reduced. She was "thrilled" that she was sleeping much better and said she was anxious to slowly wean herself off her sleep medication. At the one-month visit she also announced that she felt well enough to stop taking both antidepressants as well.

She still complained, however, of persistent constipation, severe short-term memory problems, and lack of sex drive. To address the first problem we added a magnesium citrate supplement to her program (840 mg at bedtime) and doubled the dose of the probiotic supplement (one scoop in the morning and one at bedtime). We also suspected that her intestinal flora had been greatly compromised because of her long history of medication use, so we recommended she use a one-month parasite cleansing program that contains fiber, herbs, and fructooligosaccharides (FOS), a type of short-chain sugar that supports the work of probiotics. We also recommended she significantly reduce her use of dietary sugar to help promote gut health.

For Connie's memory problems, we recommended phosphatidylserine capsules (300 mg) taken in the morning. We also believed her lack of sex drive could be remedied with an herbal and homeopathic preparation (a Life Extension formulation) and a short course of human growth hormone (0.5 IU daily six days per week). Within one month, Connie reported that her constipation had resolved completely, her energy level had increased, she was completely off her sleeping medications and was sleeping well, and her sex drive had returned.

After four months of treatment, Connie underwent another blood test, with the following results:
- DHEA-S: 428 ug/dL (65-380 ug/dL)
- Pregnenolone: 80 ng/dL (10-230 ng/dL)
- Total estrogen: 249 pg/mL (61-437 pg/mL)
- Progesterone: 5.4 ng/mL (0.2-28 ng/mL)
- Total testosterone: 62 ng/dL (14-76 ng/dL)

Even before the test results came back, Connie said, "I know my levels are good, because I feel great. I never would have believed I could feel this good again." Her husband agreed, saying his wife was feeling "999 percent better." And Connie has continued to feel great. A few months after starting treatment she decided to do a diet overhaul by eliminating processed foods and buying organic fruits and vegetables. She then added a regular walking routine to her schedule and lost five pounds, and also returned to work full-time. Today she is free of fibromyalgia, pain, fatigue, migraine, depression, and sleep problems. She also is medication-free and remains on a modification of the original hormone-restoration therapy we had suggested, along with several nutritional supplements.

In Conclusion

The basic foundation of the Migraine Cure has proven to be effective in treating and/or eliminating other significant health problems, as I've shown here. People with migraine very often also have fibromyalgia and/or high cholesterol. In the two cases presented here, the patient with fibromyalgia had migraine but considered fibromyalgia to be her primary condition, while the patient with high cholesterol did not have migraine at all, and the Migraine Cure was successful in both cases. For the woman with heart disease, a condition for which migraineurs are at increased risk, the migraine program was very effective in significantly reducing her risk for the disease.

My research and experience are showing me that the principles of the Migraine Cure, with modifications to suit each individual's specific health issue, are effective in treating other conditions as well, including obesity, erectile dysfunction, attention deficit/hyperactivity disorder, bipolar disorder, and hypocholesterolemia.

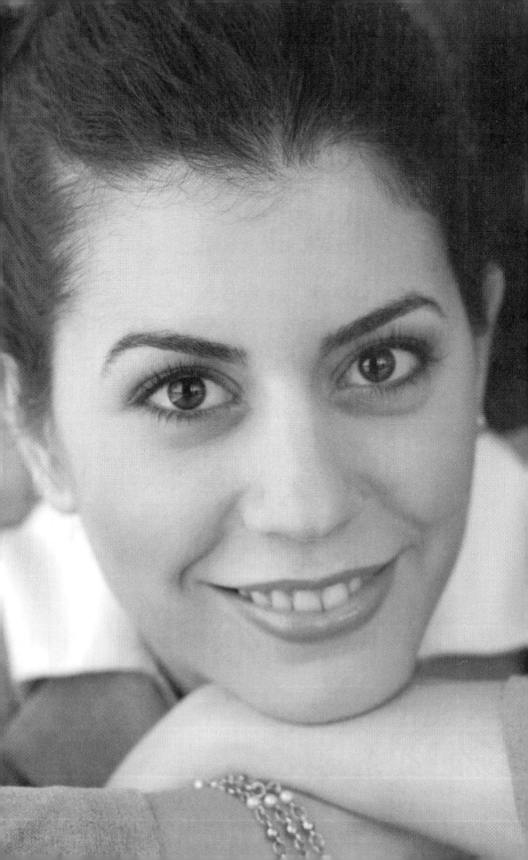

10

You Have Questions...

Q: *How long should it take for my migraines to go away once I start the Migraine Cure program?*

If you follow the recommended supplement program—including the use of bio-identical hormones—then you can expect to experience almost immediate results for some symptoms, within a day or two, with elimination of migraine within a week or so. Naturally, every person is different. Some people who have been having daily migraines find that they are headache-free the first day of the program; others get relief within a two to three days, while still others experience a significant and increasing reduction in the number and severity of their migraine headaches over several weeks until they disappear completely. In addition to how faithfully you follow the program, another factor that can impact your response includes the presence of other health problems, such as insomnia, irritable bowel, depression, anxiety, fibromyalgia, and fatigue. Remember, migraine is the result of multisystem failure. Treatment is designed to address the many interrelated systems that are out of balance and thus causing a multitude of symptoms. Each person gets back into synch at his or her own speed.

Most people are thrilled by the swiftness of their response. An example is Cory, a forty-eight-year-old dance school owner in St. Louis who began getting migraines when she was eighteen. For nearly twenty years she was experiencing three or four migraines per year, with each episode lasting three days and making her completely incapacitated. When sumatriptan

(Imitrex) was introduced to the market, she was able to better manage her migraines, and they were somewhat shorter in duration and a little less severe. At age thirty-seven she underwent a hysterectomy because of ovarian cysts, and immediately after the procedure her migraines became almost a daily occurrence. She could count on waking up with a migraine nearly every morning, but she couldn't count on sumatriptan: The relief she had once gotten with the drug disappeared. Her doctor prescribed other medications, including Elavil, Zomig, Inderal, and Celexa.

Cory noticed increasingly that her migraines were related to changes in the weather; major shifts in barometric pressure were guaranteed to trigger an episode. Alcohol was another trigger. Along with the migraine headaches, Cory experienced sleep disturbances, severe hot flashes, and loss of libido. By the time she contacted us, she was thoroughly frustrated with the poor response she was getting from her prescriptions and with her increasing fatigue. Immediately after her blood test results came back from the laboratory, she began taking the hormones and supplements we recommended.

The migraine Cory woke up with on the day she started the treatment program was the last one she would have. Along with her immediate relief from migraine came a dramatic improvement in her hot flashes. She also reported "sleeping like a baby the entire night through" after just a few days on the program, and her libido has returned.

Q: Does the Migraine Cure help eliminate other types of headache as well as migraine? I suffer with chronic tension headache nearly every day.

Although I have never *specifically* researched the effects of the Migraine Cure on people who have chronic tension headache, I can tell you this: Many people with migraine also experience daily or chronic tension headache as well, and they report that these headaches disappear, along with the migraines, when they follow the Migraine Cure.

Q: *Help! I suffer with cluster headache, and nothing seems to help. Does the Migraine Cure work for cluster headache?*

Yes, several individuals who had cluster headache have gotten complete relief when following the migraine program.

Q: *Why do you recommend that I stop taking all my supplements when I begin your treatment program? I especially don't want to stop taking calcium, because I need it for my bones.*

I can understand why you are concerned about stopping your supplement program, but this is only a temporary measure. We basically want you to begin the program with a "clean slate" and only with the supplements that are part of the program and have been chosen to help restore hormonal and metabolic balance. You can resume taking your supplements once you have restored your hormonal balance, which often takes only two to three months. Remember, the Migraine Cure involves restoration of balance in several critical systems, and restoration provides a solid foundation for health. You can get the most mileage from your supplements—including calcium--when your body is in balance.

Q: *Where can I get bio-identical estrogen?*

Although there are many patented prescription hormones available through pharmacies, sometimes getting the right combination of bio-identical estrogens can be a challenge. In particular, of the three estrogens that are recommended as part of the Migraine Cure, estriol is not currently available as a patented estrogen drug. Therefore you need to find a physician who will write you a prescription that you must fill at a compounding pharmacy. Triest® is a bio-identical, estrogen combination hormone for mula that contains estriol and is available through compounding pharmacies. Although the most common formulation of Triest is 80 percent estriol, 10 percent estradiol, and 10 percent estrone, a compounding pharmacy can create any formulation that is prescribed for you. The one I typically recommend is 90 percent estriol, 7 percent estradiol, and 3 percent estrone.

To help you find a compounding pharmacy in your area, see the "Resource" section of the Appendix, where I provide the names of several referral services and websites that have lists of compounding pharmacies.

Q: *Will my insurance cover compounded prescriptions?*

Much depends on the type of coverage you have with your insurance company. Because compounded medications do not have the National Drug Code ID numbers that manufactured drugs are required to have, some insurance companies will not reimburse compounding pharmacies directly. That means you will have to pay for the prescription in full when you pick it up. However, if you submit a claim form for your compounded medications, your insurance plan should cover the final cost and reimburse you.

Q: *Why are bio-identical hormones so important? We've been using synthetic hormones for many years.*

Bio-identical hormones are important not only for the elimination of migraine, but for overall optimal hormone balance and overall health. Synthetic hormones have a molecular structure that is unlike that of the natural hormones produced by the body, and so the body identifies these imposters as foreign material, which triggers adverse reactions, including cramps, headache, bloating, and weight gain. Even more serious is the fact that synthetic hormones increase a woman's risk of developing heart disease, stroke, dementia, and other diseases.

Bio-identical hormones, however, are exactly like those manufactured by the body, and so they are readily accepted. When we give bio-identical estrogen and progesterone, we allow the body to restore the balance between these two hormones naturally. This is good news for elimination of migraine, as well as other diseases, as I discuss in chapter 8. A balance between estrogen and progesterone also helps prevent against cancer.

Let's look at what's been happening with synthetic estrogen and hormone replacement therapy since the turn of the millennium:

- In 2001, representatives from the National Institutes of Health and the National Cancer Institute voted to place synthetic estrogen on the national list of carcinogens.
- In July 2002, the Women's Health Initiative study was halted after it was discovered that participants who were taking synthetic hormone replacement therapy (e.g., Prempro) had an increased risk of stroke, breast cancer, heart disease, and blood clots.
- In January 2003, the Food and Drug Administration (FDA) required manufacturers of synthetic estrogen and estrogen/progestin replacement therapy to include a boxed warning on their labels, informing users of the increased risks for heart attack, heart disease, breast cancer, blood clots, and stroke, and that these products are not approved for prevention of heart disease.
- In May 2003, it was reported that women older than 65 who were taking synthetic hormone replacement therapy had an increase risk of dementia or Alzheimer's disease.
- In summer 2003, several studies were published in two prestigious medical journals — the *Journal of the American Medical Association* and the *Journal of the National Cancer Institute*— in which it was revealed that women who took synthetic hormone replacement therapy had a 26 percent increased risk of breast cancer and a 54 percent increased of ovarian cancer; and

those taking synthetic estrogen replacement therapy had a 43 percent increased risk of ovarian cancer.

- In July 2005, the United Nations reclassified synthetic hormone replacement therapy from "possibly carcinogenic" to "carcinogenic."

Obviously, synthetic estrogen and estrogen/progestin replacement therapies are hazardous to your health.

Q: Is the migraine treatment program covered by insurance? How much will all of these hormones and supplements cost me?

We realize that cost can be a limiting factor for some people. Most insurance companies cover the cost of laboratory testing and hormones, but will not pay for nutritional supplements. The average total cost for three months' supply (which is the usual length of time for initial treatment) of the supplements and hormones for this program is $350. Maintenance treatment typically includes reduced doses of the hormones and only occasional use of the other supplements, as needed, so it is very possible that your insurance will pay for much of the program, including repeat blood tests as prescribed by your doctor.

Q: I read somewhere that women should not use testosterone gel, yet I see that some women who followed the Migraine Cure used this hormone. What's the story?

First let me say that testosterone is safe for women if they take it as prescribed by a knowledgeable health-care professional. That means that before anyone—female or male — takes any hormones, they should have their hormone levels evaluated. Testosterone is one of the hormones that needs to be in balance to eliminate migraine, and we recommend it only if a woman needs to restore her levels to be in balance with her other hormones. Every woman who follows the Migraine Cure program does not need to supplement with testosterone, and those who do often need to use it for only a short time. Individually compounded, low-dose testosterone supplements are available in gel as well as a transdermal patch, capsule, and tablets. I recommend the gel because a compounding pharmacist can create the exact formula for a patient's needs, and it is easy to use.

Q: You make very specific recommendations for each of the hormones and supplements in your treatment program. Is it necessary for me to use these specific brands, or can I make appropriate substitutions?

The hormones and supplements that I recommend for the treatment program were selected after much careful testing and evaluation and were chosen because they provided the best results. The most important things to remember when you choose the hormones and supplements for this treatment program is that the hormones must be bio-identical, and all the supplements should be from reputable, high-quality manufacturers. After all, you want results, and you can only get results if you follow the dosing recommendations and the products you buy contain the potency they advertise. Therefore, for example, you can bypass the melatonin product recommended in the program and purchase melatonin, kava root extract, and vitamin B6 in a way that provides you with the same quality and quantity found in the recommended product.

Q: I, like many other migraineurs, have fibromyalgia. Why do these two conditions occur together so often?

I have found that about 17 percent of migraineurs also have fibromyalgia. The good news, however, is that the Migraine Cure can completely eliminate this syndrome as well. Some doctors believe the main cause of fibromyalgia is an irreversible disturbance of the neuroimmunoendocrinological system, a complex relationship that involves the nervous system, the immune system, and the endocrine glands. We partially agree with this hypothesis, in that we believe that individuals who have this syndrome have a dysfunction of the autonomic nervous system caused by hormonal deficiency that is associated with an inability of the cell membranes to respond appropriately to hormonal impulses. We do not agree, however, that fibromyalgia is irreversible, because we have seen the condition disappear in patients who have received hormone restoration. My belief is that, like migraine, fibromyalgia is the result of a loss of balance within the neurohormonal and metabolic systems. Once we restore balance in those systems, as we do in the Migraine Cure, fibromyalgia, like migraine, disappears.

Several factors support the idea that migraine and fibromyalgia share a common physiologic abnormality. One is the fact that fibromyalgia (like migraine) primarily affects women, especially during their reproductive years, which suggests a relationship between fibromyalgia and sex hormones. Reduced fertility and delayed menstruation, both common in fibromyalgia, may be signs of a hormone imbalance. Another is the fact that characteristics of fibromyalgia—musculoskeletal pain, chronic fatigue, gastrointestinal problems, sleep disturbances, and psychological disorders—are similar to those seen in people who have hormonal deficiencies, as well as in people who have migraine. Yet another factor is that disruption of the hypothalamic-pituitary-adrenal (HPA) axis, which I discussed in chapter 2, is characteristic of both fibromyalgia and migraine. Low levels of melatonin, which cause sleep disturbances, also are seen in both fibromyalgia and migraine patients. Again, we are fortunate that melatonin supplementation is effective against the pain, depression, and sleep problems experienced by these patients.

Q: *How long will I have to keep taking the different hormones and supplements that are part of your migraine program?*

The bio-identical hormone dosages recommended as part of the Migraine Cure are designed to restore your hormones to "youthful" levels, those that adults reach between the ages of 20 and 29. Remember that two of the hormones, pregnenolone and DHEA, are precursors for the other steroid hormones that are also part of the Migraine Cure. That being said, when a migraineur who is younger than 35 years participates in the Migraine Cure, we usually recommend that he or she take the suggested bio-identical hormones for at least three months. That's because it appears that the hormone function of the body of a younger individual re-sets itself when these two supplemental hormones are given. Therefore these individuals typically can gradually stop taking the hormone supplements.

Among older adults, however, supplemental bio-identical hormones are recommended for a lifetime. When you keep your hormones at an optimal level (optimal for your own specific needs), you'll feel great overall and also know that you are fighting against aging as well. This is true for everyone, not just individuals who have migraine. In fact, as you've seen in chapter 8, achieving balanced hormone levels is critical when it comes to successfully treating other serious medical conditions, including fibromyalgia, high cholesterol, and coronary heart disease.

We usually suggest that individuals take melatonin and kava root extract whenever they have problems with sleep or if they are going through an especially stressful or anxious period in their lives. Probiotics also can be used intermittently, usually for one month at a time, if you experience some gastrointestinal problems or especially if you need to take antibiotics for any reason. If you are like most Americans, you are deficient in magnesium, and so you may need to continue taking magnesium as well. Saw palmetto is recommended for anyone who is taking hormones, because it blocks conversion of testosterone to DHT, thus helping to prevent the development of prostate enlargement and hair loss. This herb also helps prevent bladder inflammation and supports bladder health in women, an important consideration as women age because they tend to experience some loss of bladder control, resulting in urinary incontinence.

Q: Do you recommend a specific diet or eating plan as part of your Migraine Cure?

Although I firmly believe that a whole foods, toxin-free diet is the healthiest approach for everyone, migraineur or not, I do not emphasize a specific eating plan as part of the Migraine Cure. And here's why. Migraineurs typically have had to eliminate many things from their lives, including foods, beverages, and activities other people enjoy. The goal of the Migraine Cure is to allow people to return to a NORMAL, healthy life. Once they are free of migraine and its related symptoms, people find they are free to enjoy chocolate, alcoholic beverages, and other food items that used to trigger their pain. Naturally, I believe everything should be done in moderation: I am not advocating excessive use of alcohol or any type of food or beverage. When former migraineurs have "gotten their groove back," as one former patient calls it, I highly recommend they adopt healthy eating habits, and that includes incorporating as many whole, organic fruits, vegetables, grains, nuts, and beans in their diet as possible, along with organic meats and dairy products and safe fish choices as they choose. I also strongly suggest they always eat breakfast, make lunch the largest meal of the day, and always leave at least four hours between dinner and bedtime.

Q: Why don't you recommend stress management or relaxation techniques as part of the Migraine Cure? Isn't stress reduction important for eliminating migraine?

I absolutely believe stress reduction is important, but until you restore the foundation of your health—which is accomplished through hormone restoration therapy, probiotics, resetting the pineal gland, and rebalancing magnesium and calcium, it is impossible to control stress on a permanent basis. Indeed, many people find that as soon as they are migraine-free, their energy increases, and their other symptoms fall away one by one, they are eager to adopt new activities or return to ones they once enjoyed, including exercise, going to the gym, yoga, tai chi, meditation, and other things individuals say are relaxing and enjoyable for them. You certainly are free to include relaxation techniques as part of your program when you begin the Migraine Cure, but I do not emphasize it as part of the general plan.

Q: *I'm a "graduate" of your Migraine Cure, and I feel great! I've been migraine-free for more than a year now. But occasionally I still experience some sleep problems, like waking up and not being able to go back to sleep. I know I can take melatonin whenever I feel I need it, but are there any other natural ways to deal with this intermittent problem?*

I'm glad to hear that you're feeling great. Yes, you can take melatonin, which helps restore dominance of your parasympathetic nervous system at night. I don't know how much you were taking before, but the usual dose is from 0.5 to 6 mg 30 minutes before bedtime.

You can also consider kava root extract, which, if you were following our recommendations, is part of the Migraine Cure program. Other supplements that are effective in relieving insomnia and insomniac mood disorders include St. John's Wort, choline, omega-3 fatty acids, B complex vitamins, and SAM-e. Some people find that a cup of chamomile tea taken before bedtime is helpful for mild insomnia. For more persistent or severe insomnia, valerian root appears to be as effective as some prescription medications. Valerian makes falling asleep easier and helps the body enter a deeper sleep state. A dose of 400 mg 30 minutes before bedtime is usually effective.

Some other tips to help you get a restful night sleep include:
- Avoid consuming any stimulating beverages, supplements, or medications late in the day; for example, caffeine, nicotine, alcohol, ginseng, guarana, ashwaganda.

- Avoid taking naps during the day. If you really need to take a nap, make it a twenty-minute one.
- Do not eat a large meal in the evening. Strive to make lunch your biggest meal of the day.
- Exercise regularly, but do not exercise within two to three hours of bedtime.
- Spend some time doing relaxation or stress-reduction techniques before bedtime. This may include a warm bath, meditation, breathing exercises, or listening to soothing music.

Q: I see you use kava kava as part of your program to restore balance to the pineal gland. Hasn't kava been linked with liver damage?

If you take megadoses of *any* supplement, you run the risk of liver toxicity or other potentially dangerous side effects. As I explain in chapter 5, kava got some bad press as the result of *one* study conducted in Germany, and a poorly conducted and erroneously reported study at that. While it is true that some of the people in the study developed liver disease, what the reports did *not* reveal is that most of the participants who had cirrhosis, hepatitis, or were on dialysis were taking more than ten times the normal dose of kava daily; our recommendation is 250 mg daily, while these patients were taking 4,000 mg or more. Also, some of the individuals regularly used alcohol (which is known to damage the liver), and most of the patients were taking at least one prescription medication, which can increase the possibility of liver damage as well.

In addition to the responsible dose recommended in the Migraine Cure, patients typically take kava and melatonin for a very short time—until their migraine is gone, which is usually within two to four weeks of starting supplementation. After that, they may use kava root extract occasionally and briefly, for one or two days as needed. Then, as an added precaution, we also recommend that individuals have their blood rechecked for hormone levels and liver and kidney function after they have been following the treatment program for a month or two, and then again after about four months. We are always mindful of the first rule of medicine: "Do no harm."

Q: *I've read that pregnenolone should not be taken by anyone who has a hormone-related cancer, yet you recommend pregnenolone as part of your migraine program. Should I be concerned about pregnenolone if I have cancer or am at high-risk for a hormone-related cancer?*

Migraineurs in general, including those who participate in the Migraine Cure, are usually deficient in pregnenolone. The pregnenolone we recommend for these individuals is designed to restore their pregnenolone and related hormones to youthful, healthy levels, not elevate them to dangerous, unhealthy ones. People who have hormone-related cancer, such as prostate cancer and estrogen-receptor positive breast cancer, or individuals who are at high risk of such cancers do not have to be concerned about taking pregnenolone as part of the Migraine Cure. Remember: only when your hormones are in balance can you hope to stave off major health problems.

Q: *I am currently taking synthetic progestins and want to switch to natural progesterone. I noticed there's a big difference in the dosages; for example, I was taking 5 mg of progestin, and it looks like I'm supposed to take at least 50 mg of progesterone? Is that right? Why the big difference in dosages?*

I'm glad you have decided to switch to natural progesterone and hope you are balancing all of your hormones by using bio-identical products! When it comes to progesterone and progestin, synthetic progestins are ten to one hundred times as potent as natural progesterone. Therefore, if you were

taking 5 mg of synthetic progestin, an equivalent amount of natural progesterone would be 50 to 500 mg, depending on your specific needs.

Q: *The first time I took probiotics, my stomach bothered me, so I stopped taking them. Why did I have that reaction?*

Probiotics are "good" bacteria, and when they enter the gut they help
eliminate the "bad," toxic bacteria. Depending on how toxic your gut is,
the actual process of the bacteria "dying off" may cause some temporary
side effects, such as bloating, gas, and headache. These symptoms are only
temporary and are a common occurrence when the body is ridding itself of
toxins. Start taking the probiotics again, and after a day or two you should
feel much better.

Q: *In several cases you recommended a one-month parasite cleansing treatment. What do parasites have to do with migraine?*

More than 90 percent of Americans have parasites residing in their gut,
brain, blood, muscle, and other parts of their body. Parasites can come
from various sources, including pets, exposure to contaminated soil, trav-
eling to foreign countries (especially South America), and inadequately prepared foods. We have found that some individuals continue to experience
fatigue or to have difficulties with intestinal health, even after they have
been following the treatment program for a month or longer. That's when
we suspect parasites may be the cause, and so we recommend a mild, one-
month parasite-cleansing program, and the results are typically excellent. In
such cases, eliminating parasites is part of the digestive restoration portion
of the program.

Source Notes

CHAPTER 1

Bauer AW. Between symbol and symptom: pain and its meanings in classical antiquity. *Schmerz* 1996 Aug 26; 10(4): 169-75.

Beckett BE, Herndon KC. Headache Disorders. In Dipiro JT, Talbert RL et al., eds. Pharmacotherapy: *A Pathophysiologic Approach*. McGraw-Hill Companies, Inc.; 2002 Jan 1: 5(61):1119-35.

Bigal ME et al. New migraine preventive options: an update with pathophysiological considerations. *Rev Hosp Clin* 2002; 57(6).

Breslau N et al. Comorbidity of migraine and depression: investigating potential etiology and prognosis. *Neurology* 2003 April 22; 60(8): 1308-12.

Cassidy EM, et al. Central 5-HT receptor hypersensitivity in migraine without aura. *Cephalalgia*. 2003 Feb;23(1):29-34.

Claustrat B, et al. Nocturnal plasma melatonin levels in migraine: a preliminary report. *Headache* 1989 Apr; 29(4):242-45.

Claustrat B, Brun J, et al. Nocturnal plasma melatonin profile and melatonin kinetics during infusion in status migrainosus. *Cephalalgia* 1997 Jun; 17(4):511-17.

Colson NJ et al. The role of vascular and hormonal genes in migraine susceptibility. *Mol Genet Metab* 2006 Jan 3.

Estevez M, Gardner KL. Update on the genetics of migraine. *Hum Genet* 2004 Feb; 114(3): 225-35.

Etminan M et al. Risk of ischemic stroke in people with migraine: systemic review and meta-analysis of observational studies. *Br Med J* 2005 Jan 8; 330(7482):63.

Gagnier JJ. The therapeutic potential of melatonin in migraines and other headache types. *Altern Med Rev* 2001 Aug; 6(4):383- 89.

Gelmers HJ. Calcium-channel blockers in the treatment of migraine. *Am J Cardiol* 1985 Jan 25; 55(3):139B-43B.

Joubert J. Diagnosing headache. *Aust Fam Physician* 2005 Aug; 34(8):621-5.

Kasper DL, Braunwald DE. et al. *Harrison's Principles of Internal Medicine*. 16.ed. New York: McGraw-Hill Professional, 2005.

Koehler PJ, Isler H. The early use of ergotamine in migraine. Edward Woakes' report of 1868, its theoretical and practical background and its international reception. *Cephalalgia* 2002 Oct; 22(8):686-91

Kors EE et al. Recent findings in headache genetics. *Curr Opin Neurol* 2004 Jun; 17(3): 283-88.

Kurth T et al. Migraine, headache, and the risk of stroke in women: a prospective study. *Neurology* 2005 Mar 22; 64(6): 1020-26.

Lipton RB et al. Prevalence and burden of migraine in the United States: results from the American Migraine Study II. *Headache* 2001; 41:646-57.

Lipton RB, Stewart WF, Simon D. Medical consultation for migraine: results from the American Migraine Study. *Headache* 1998; 38:87-96.

Lipton RB, Scher AI, et al: Migraine in the United States. *Neurology* 58:885, 2002.
Lipton R, Stewart WF. Migraine in the United

States: a review of epidemiology and health care use. *Neurology* 1993; 43:S6-S10.

MacGregor EA, Chia H, Vohrah RC, et al. Migraine and menstruation: a pilot study. *Cephalalgia* 1990; 10(6):305-10.

Martin VT, Behbehani MM: Toward a rational understanding of migraine trigger factors. *Med Clin North Am* 85:911, 2001.

Merck Manual: www.merckmedicus.com/pp/us/hcp/disease-modules/migraine/pathophysiology_sub.jsp

National Institute of Neurological Disorders and Stroke; www.ninds.nih.gov/

Sargeant L et al. Headache, Cluster. March 10, 2005; article at www.emedicine.com/EMERG/topic229.htm

Selmaj K. Blood serotonin level in sciatica and the serotonin theory of migraine pathogenesis. *Neurol Neurochir Pol* 1979 Mar; 13(2):169-72.

Silberstein SD, Young WB. Headache and Facial Pain. In: Goetz CG, Eds. *Textbook of Clinical Neurology*. Philadelphia: Elsevier Science (USA); 2003 Jan 1: 2(53):1187-206.

Stewart WF et al. Prevalence of migraine in the United States: relation to age, income, race, and other sociodemographic factors. *JAMA* 1992; 267(1): 64-69.

Thomas Jefferson University website http://www.tju.edu/headache/info/index.cfm

Toglia JU. Melatonin: a significant contributor to the pathogenesis of migraine. *Med Hypotheses*. 2001 Oct; 57(4):432-34.

Toglia JU. Is migraine due to a deficiency of pineal melatonin? *Ital J Neurol Sci* 1986 Jun; 7(3):319-23.

Welch KM, D'Andrea G, et al. The concept of migraine as a state of central neuronal hyperexcitability. *Neurol Clin* 1990 Nov; 8(4):817-28.

Welch KM. Brain hyperexcitability: The basis for antiepileptic drugs in migraine prevention. *Headache: The Journal of Head and Face Pain* Apr 2005; 45(1): S25-S32.

Welch KM. Pathogenesis of migraine. *Semin Neurol* 1997; 17(4):335-41.

CHAPTER 2

Blakeslee, Sandra. Complex and hidden brain in gut makes bellyaches and butterflies. New York Times, January 23, 1996; article at http://aikidoaus.com.au/dojo/docs/2nd_braina.htm

Bock, Kenneth and Nellie Saben. *The Road to Immunity*. New York: Simon & Schuster/Pocket, 1997.

Claustrat B, et al. Nocturnal plasma melatonin levels in migraine: a preliminary report. *Headache* 1989 Apr; 29(4):242-5;

Claustrat B, Brun J, et al. Nocturnal plasma melatonin profile and melatonin kinetics during infusion in status migrainosus. *Cephalalgia* 1997 Jun; 17(4):511-7;

Epstein MT, Hockaday JM, Hockaday TD. Migraine and reproductive hormones throughout the menstrual cycle. *Lancet* 1975; 1:543-48.

Facchinetti F et al. Reduced testosterone levels in cluster headache: a stress-related phenomenon? *Cephalalgia* 1986; 6:29-34.

Gagnier JJ. The therapeutic potential of melatonin in migraines and other headache types. *Altern Med Rev* 2001 Aug; 6(4):383- 9.

Kasper DL, Braunwald DE. et al. *Harrison's Principles of Internal Medicine. 16.ed.* New York: McGraw-Hill Professional, 2005.

Peres MF et al. Melatonin, 3 mg is effective for migraine prevention. *Neurology* 2004 Aug 24; 63(4): 757.

Pharmacy Times. Serotonin is important in gut function. Article at www.pharmacytimes.com/article.cfm?ID=355

Romili A et al. Low plasma testosterone levels in cluster headache. *Cephalalgia* 1983; 3:41-46.

Toglia JU. Melatonin: a significant contributor to the pathogenesis of migraine. *Med Hypotheses* 2001 Oct; 57(4):432-4;

Toglia JU. Is migraine due to a deficiency of pineal melatonin? *Ital J Neurol Sci* 1986 Jun; 7(3):319-23.

Waldenlind E, Gustafsson SA. Prolactin in cluster headache: diurnal secretion, response to thyrotropin-releasing hormone, and relation to sex steroids and gonadotropins. *Cephalalgia* 1987; 7:43-54.

CHAPTER 3

Campagnoli C et al. Progestins and progesterone in hormone replacement therapy and the risk of breast cancer. *J Steroid Biochem Mol Biol* 2005 Jul; 96(2): 95-108.

Beasley, Deena. Study says pivotal hormone therapy trial was flawed. December 16, 2005; see Reuters article at http://www.somersetmedicalcenter.com/118127.cfm

Chlebowski RT et al. Influence of estrogen and progestin on breast cancer and mammography in healthy postmenopausal women. *JAMA* 2003; 289:3243-53.

Gobel H, et al. Comparison of naratriptan and sumatriptan in recurrence-prone migraine patients. Naratriptan International Recurrence Study Group. *Clin Ther* 2000 Aug; 22 (8): 981-89.

Gobel H, et al. Open-labeled long- term study of the efficacy, safety, and tolerability of subcutaneous sumatriptan in acute migraine treatment. *Cephalalgia* 1999 Sep; 19(7):676-83.

Kasper DL, Braunwald DE. et al. *Harrison's Principles of Internal Medicine.* 16.ed. New York: McGraw-Hill Professional, 2005.

Klaiber EL, Vogel W, Rako S. A critique of the Women's Health Initiative hormone therapy study. *Fert Steril* Dec. 2005; 84(96): 1589-1601.

Lake AE 3rd, Saper JR. Chronic headache: New advances in treatment strategies. *Neurology* 2002 Sep 10; 59(5 Suppl 2):S8- 13.

Lawrence EC. Diagnosis and management of migraine headaches. *South Med J* 2004 Nov; 97(11):1069-77

MacGregor EA. Is HRT giving you a headache? *British Migraine Association Newsletter* 1993, pp 19-24.

Melhado E et al. Headache during pregnancy in women with a prior history of menstrual headaches. *Arq Neuro-Psiquiatr* 2005 Dec; 63(4).

Rapoport AM. Frovatriptan: pharmacological

differences and clinical results. *Curr Med Res Opin* 2001; 17 Suppl 1:s68-70.

Silberstein SD, Lipton RB. Overview of diagnosis and treatment of migraine. *Neurology* 1994 Oct; 44(10 Suppl 7):S6-16.

Silberstein SD. Practice parameter: evidence-based guidelines for migraine headache (an evidence-based review): report of the Quality Standards Subcommittee of the American Academy of Neurology. *Neurology* 2000 Sep 26; 55(6):754-62.

Stein DG. The case for progesterone. *Ann NY Acad Sci* 2005 Jun; 1052:152-69.

Writing Group for the Women's Health Initiative Investigators. Risks and benefits of estrogen plus progestin in healthy post-menopausal women. Principal results from the Women's Health Initiative randomized control trial. *JAMA* 2002; 288(3):321-33.

Young WB, Hopkins MM, Shechter AL, Silberstein SD. Topiramate: a case series study in migraine prophylaxis. *Cephalalgia* 2002 Oct; 22(8):659-63.

CHAPTER 4

American Heart Association website: www.americanheart.org/presenter.jhtml?identifier=183

Araghi-Niknam, M, et al. Dehydroepiandrosterone (DHEA) sulfate prevents reduction in tissue vitamin E and increased lipid peroxidation due to murine retrovirus infection of aged mice. *Proc Soc Exp Biol Med* 1998 Jul; 218(3): 210-7.

Barrett-Connor, E et al. Endogenous levels of dehydroepiandrosterone sulfate, but not other sex hormones, are associated with depressed mood in older women: the Rancho Bernardo Study. *J Am Geriatr Soc* 1999 Jun; 47(6): 685-91.

Baulieu EE, Thomas G, et al. Dehydroepiandrosterone (DHEA), DHEA sulfate, and aging: contribution of the DHEAge Study to a sociobiomedical issue. *Proc Natl Acad Sci* USA 2000 Apr 11; 97(8):4279-84.

Cutolo, M. Sex hormone adjuvant therapy in rheumatoid arthritis. *Rheum Dis Clin North Am* 2000; 26: 881-95.

Dalton K. *The Premenstrual Syndrome and*

Progesterone Therapy. Chicago: Year Book Medical Publishers, 1977.

Dalton K. *Once a Month.* Pomona CA: Hunter, 1979.

Evans RW, Mathew NT. *Handbook of Headache.* Philadelphia: Lippincott-Williams & Wilkins, 2000; excerpt at website: www.migraines.org/treatment/treather.htm

Hargrove JT et al. Menopausal hormone replacement therapy with continuous daily oral micronized estradiol and progesterone. *Obstetrics & Gynecology* 71:606-12, 1989.

Head KA. Estriol: safety and efficacy. *Altern Med Rev* 1998 Apr; 3(2): 101-13.

Hotze SF. *Hormones, Health, and Happiness.* Houston: Forrest Publishing, 2005.

Pete Hueseman, RPh, PD. Synthetic progestins and natural progesterone. A pharmacist explores the differences. Article at: http://www.project-aware.org/Resource/articlearchives/differences.shtml

Jesse, RL et al. Dehydroepiandrosterone inhibits human platelet aggregation in vitro and in vivo. *Ann NY Acad* Sci 1995 Dec 29; 774: 281-90.

Khorram, O. et al. Activation of immune function by dehydroepiandrosterone (DHEA) in age-advanced men. *J Gerontol A Biol Sci Med Sci* 1997 Jan; 52(1): M1-M7.

Legrain S, Massien C, et al. Dehydroepiandrosterone replacement administration: pharmacokinetic and pharmacodynamic studies in healthy elderly subjects. *J Clin Endocrinol Metab* 2000 Sep; 85(9):3208-17.

Lemon HM. Oestriol and prevention of breast cancer. *The Lancet* March 10, 1973: 546-47.

Li R et al. *Proceedings of the National Academy of Sciences*, December 19, 2005.

Lichten EM, et al. The confirmation of a biochemical marker for women's hormonal migraine: the depo-estradiol challenge test. *Headache* 1996; 36(6): 367-70.

Li W et al. Sex steroid hormones exert biphasic effects on cytosolic magnesium ions in cerebral vascular smooth muscle cells: possible relationships to migraine frequency in premenstrual syndromes and stroke incidence. *Brain Res Bull* 2001 Jan 1:54(1): 83-89.

Morales AJ, et al. Effects of replacement dose of dehydroepiandrosterone in men and women of advancing age. *J Clin Endocrinol Metab* 1994; 78:1360-67.

Oberbeck, R et al. Dehydroepiandrosterone decreases mortality rate and improves cellular immune function during polymicrobial sepsis. *Crit Care Med* 2001 Feb; 29(2):380-4.

O'Shaughnessy A, et al. Circulating divalent cations in asymptomatic ovarian hyperstimulation and in vitro fertilization patients. *Gynecol Obstet Invest* 2001; 52(4): 237-42.

Partonen T et al. Association of low serum total cholesterol with major depression and suicide. *Br J Psychiatry* 1999 Sep; 175: 259-62.

Silberstein SD, Merriam GR. Sex hormones and headache. In Goadsby PJ, Silberstein SD. *Headache*. Boston, Butterworth-Heinemann, 1997, pp 143-176.

Straub, RH, Scholmerich, J, Zietz, B. Replacement therapy with DHEA plus corticosteroids in patients with chronic inflammatory diseases-substitutes of adrenal and sex hormones. Z. *Rheumatol.* 2000; 59(Suppl. 2): II/108-18 (in German).

Suarez E. Relations of trait depression and anxiety to low lipid and lipoprotein concentrations in healthy young adult women. *Psychosomatic Med* May-June 1999; 61(3): 273-79.

Tolsa JF, Gao Y, Raj JU. Developmental change in magnesium sulfate-induced relaxation of rabbic pulmonary arteries. *J Appl Physiol* 1999 Nov; 87(5): 1589-94.

Wolkowitz, OM et al. Dehydroepiandrosterone (DHEA) treatment of depression. *Biol Psychiatry* 1997 Feb 1; 41(3): 311-8.

CHAPTER 5

Alvarez GG, Ayas NT. The impact of daily sleep duration on health: A review of the literature. *Prog Cardiovasc Nurs.* 2004 Spring; 19(2): 56-59 The impact of daily sleep duration on health: a review of the literature. *Prog Cardiovasc Nurs.* 2004 Spring; 19(2):56-59.

Avas NT, White DP, et al. A prospective study of self-reported sleep duration and incident diabetes in women. *Diabetes Care.* 2003 Feb;26(2):380-84.

Avas NT, White, DP et al. A prospective study of sleep duration and coronary heart disease in women. *Arch Intern Med.* 2003 Jan 27;163(2):205-9.

Bellipanni G, et al. Effects of melatonin in perimenopausal and menopausal women: our personal experience. *Ann N Y Acad Sci* 2005 Dec; 1057: 393-402.

Brush MG et al. Pyridoxine in the treatment of premenstrual syndrome: a retrospective survey in 630 patients. *Br J Clin Pract* 1988 Nov; 42(11): 448-52.

Cagnacci A et al. Prolonged melatonin administration decreases nocturnal blood pressure in women. *Am J Hypertens* 2005 Dec; 18(12 Pt 1):1614-18.

Cajochen C et al. Role of melatonin in the regulation of human circadian rhythms and sleep. *J neuroendocrinology* 2003; 15:432-37.

Citera G et al. The effect of melatonin in patients with fibromyalgai: a pilot study. *Clin Rheumatol* 2000; 19(1): 9-13.

Claustrat B, Brun J, et al. Melatonin secretion is supersensitivity to light in migraine. *Cephalalgia* 2004 Feb; 24(2): 128-33.

Clouatre DL. Kava kava: examining new reports of toxicity. *Toxicol Lett* 2004 Apr. 15; 150(1): 85-96.

DeLeo V et al. Evaluation of combining kava extract with hormone replacement therapy in the treatment of postmenopausal anxiety. *Maturitas* 2001 Aug 25; 39(2): 185-88.

DeLeo V et al. Assessment of the association of kava-kava extract and hormone replacement therapy in the treatment of postmenopause anxiety. *Minerva Ginecol* 2000 Jun; 52(6): 263-67.

Diegoli MS. A double-blind trial of four medications to treat severe premenstrual syndrome. *Int J Gynaecol Obstet* 1998 Jul; 62(1):63-67.

Eli R, Fasciano JA. A chronopharmacological preventive treatment for sleep-related migraine headaches and chronic morning headaches: nitric oxide supersensitivity can cause sleep-related headaches in a subset of patients. *Med Hypotheses* 2006; 66(3): 461-65.

Fernandez B et al. Relationship between adenohypophyseal and steroid hormones and variations in serum and urinary melatonin levels during the ovarian cycle, perimenopause and menopause in healthy women. *J Steroid Biochem* 1990 Feb; 35(2): 257-62.

Gagnier JJ. The therapeutic potential of melatonin in migraines and other headache types. *Altern Med Rev* 2001 Aug; 6(4): 383-89.

Geier FP, Konstantinowicz T. Kava treatment in patients with anxiety. *Phytother Res* 2004 Apr; 18(4): 297-300

Gilad E. et al. Melatonin inhibits expression of the inducible isoform of nitric oxide synthase in murine macrophages. *FASEB J* 1998; 12:685-93.

Heslop P, Smith GD, et al. Sleep duration and mortality: The effect of short or long sleep duration on cardiovascular and all-cause mortality in working men and women. *Sleep Med.* 2002 Jul;3(4):305-14;

Kelman L. High prevalence of migraine triggers. *Neurology Reviews* 13(10); Oct. 2005, at http://www.neurologyreviews.com/oct05/MigraineTriggers.html

Lambert, Geoff and Dr. Alessandro Zagami, Department of Neurology, Prince Henry Hospital, at http://www.brainaustralia.org.au/research/report_on_2002_reasearchprojects/how_does_migraine_treatment_work

Lehrl S. Clinical efficacy of kava extract WS 1490 in sleep disturbances associated with anxiety disorders. Results of a multicenter, randomized placebo-controlled, double-blind clinical trial. *J Affect Disord* 2004 Dec; 83 (2-3): 287.

Leone M, D'Amico D, et al. Melatonin versus placebo in the prophylaxis of cluster headache: a double-blind pilot study with parallel groups. *Cephalalgia* 1996; 16:494–96.

Lu WZ, Gwee KA, Moochhalla S, Ho KY. Melatonin improves bowel symptoms in female patients with irritable bowel syndrome: a double-blind placebo-controlled study. *Aliment Pharmacol Ther* 2005 Nov 15; 22(10): 927-34.

Mack, Kenneth MD. Presentation at the Annual Conference on Sleep Disorders in Infants and Childhood, January 2006.

Nagtegaal JE, Smits MG, Swart ACW, et al. Melatonin-responsive headache in delayed sleep phase syndrome: preliminary observations. *Headache* 1998; 38:303–7.

Nitric oxide: From menace to marvel of the decade. A briefing document prepared for the Royal Society and Association of British Science Writers. May 1996, at www.absw. org.uk/ Briefings/Nitric%20oxide.htm

Peres FP et al. Melatonin, 3 mg, is effective for migraine prevention. *Neurology* 2004 Aug; 63:757.

PittlerMH, Ernst E. Kava extract for treating anxiety. *Cochrane Database Syst Rev* 2002; (2): CD003393

Rist, Curtis. The pain is in the brain—migraines. Quoting Jes Olesen, MD. Discover March 2000. At http://www.findarticles.com/p/articles/mi_m1511/is_3_21/ai_59535401/pg_2

Scheer FA et al. Daily nighttime melatonin reduces blood pressure in male patients with essential hypertension. *Hypertension* 2004 Feb; 43(2):192-97.

Song GH, Leng PH, et al. Melatonin supplementation may help relieve abdominal pain in patients with IBS. *Gut* 2005; 54(10): 1402-7.

Weibel L, Follenius M, Brandenberger G. Biologic rhythms: their changes in night-shift workers. *Presse Med* 1999 Feb 6; 28(5):252-58.

Toglia JU. Is migraine due to a deficiency of pineal melatonin? *Ital J Neurol Sci* (ITALY) Jun 1986; 7(3): 319-23.

CHAPTER 6

Blakeslee, Sandra. Complex and hidden brain in gut makes bellyaches and butterflies. *New York Times,* January 23, 1996; at http://aikidoaus.com.au/dojo/docs/2nd_braina. htm

Bouhnik Y, Flourie B, et al. Administration of transgalacto-oligosaccharides increases fecal bifidobacteria and modifies colonic fermentation metabolism in healthy humans. *J Nutr* 1997;127:444-8.

Bhounik Y, et al. Short-chain fructo-oligosaccharide administration dose-dependently increases fecal bifidobacteria in healthy humans. *J Nutr* 1999;129:113-16.

Davidson MH, Synecki C, Maki KC, Drennen KB. Effects of dietary inulin in serum lipids in men and women with hypercholesterolaemia. *Nutr Res* 1998; 3:503-17.

Delzenne NM. The hypolipidaemic effect of inulin: when animal studies help to approach the human problem. *Br J Nutr* 1999; 82:3-4.

Jackson KG, et al. The effect of the daily intake of inulin on fasting lipid, insulin and glucose concentrations in middle-aged men and women. *Br J Nutr* 1999; 82:23-30.

Kalliomaki M, et al. Probiotics in primary prevention of atopic disease: a randomized placebo-controlled trial. *Lancet* 2001; 357: 1076-1079.

Kankaanpaa P, et al. Dietary fatty acids and allergy. *Ann Med* 1999; 31: 282-287.

Kirjavainen PV, Apostolou E, Salminen SJ, Isolaure E. New aspects of probiotics – a novel approach in the management of food allergy. *Allergy* 1999; 54: 909-15.

Kumar D, Thompson PD, Wingate DL et al. Abnormal REM sleep in the irritable bowel syndrome. *Gastroenterology*. 1992 Jul; 103(1):12-17

Laiho K, Hoppu U, et al. Probiotics: on-going research on atopic individuals. *Br J Nutr* 2002; 88 (suppl)1: S19-S27.

Majamaa H, Isolauri E. Probiotics: a novel approach in the management of food allergy. *J Allergy Clin Immunol* 1997; 99: 175-185.

Mayer E, MD. Quoted in article on Blue Cross/Blue Shield website at www.ahealthyme. com/article/primer/101186767

Millichap JG, Yee MM. The diet factor in pediatric and adolescent migraine. *Pediatr Neurol* 2003 Jan; 28(1): 9-15.

Mulak A, Paradowsk L. Migraine and irritable bowel syndrome. *Neurol Neurochir Pol* 2005; 39(4 Suppl 1): S55-60.

Nahas Z et al. Two-year outcome of vagus nerve stimulation (VNS) for treatment of major depressive episodes. J Clin Psychiatry 2005 Sep; 66(9): 1097-1104.

Pelton, Ross. Interview in *Life Extension Magazine* at http://www.lef.org/magazine/mag 2000/dec2000_interview.html

Plummer N, Wood C. The neonatal immune system and risk of allergy a delicate balancing act, positively influenced by probiotics and fatty acids. *Townsend Letter for Doctors and Patients*, Feb-March 2002; 94-105.

Roberfroid MB, Van Loo JAE, Gibson GR. The bifidogenic nature of chicory inulin and its hydrolysis products. *J Nutr* 1998; 128:11-19.

Roberfroid M. Dietary fibre, inulin and oligofructose. A review comparing their physiological effects. *Crit Rev Food Sci Nutr* 1993; 33:103-48.

Schultz V. Hansel R, Tyler VE. Rational Phytotherapy. *A Physician's Guide to Herbal Medicine.* Berlin: Springer-Verlag, 1998.

Song GH, Leng RH, et al. Melatonin improves abdominal pain in irritable bowel syndrome patients who have sleep disturbances: a randomized, double-blind, placebo controlled study. *Gut* 2005; 54(10): 1402-7.

Weiss RF, Fintelmann V. *Herbal Medicine*, 2nd ed. Stuttgart: Thieme, 2000.

Yamashita K, Kawai K, Itakura M. Effect of fructo-oligosaccharides on blood glucose and serum lipids in diabetic subjects. *Nutr Res* 1984;4:961-66.

CHAPTER 7

Aloisi P, Marrelli A, Porto C, Tozzi E, Cerone G. Visual evoked potentials and serum magnesium levels in juvenile migraine patients. *Headache* 1997 Jun;37(6):383-5.

Bigal ME et al. Intravenous magnesium sulphate in the acute treatment of migraine without aura and migraine with aura. A randomized, double-blind, placebo-controlled study. *Cephalalgia* 2002 Jun; 22(5): 345-53.

Elin R: Assessment of magnesium status. *Clin Chem.* 33:1965-1970, 1987.

Elisaf M, Bairaktari E, Kalaitzidis R, Siamopoulos K. Hypomagnesemia in alcoholic patients. *Alcohol Clin Exp Res* 1998; 22:244-46.

Ford ES and Mokdad AH. Dietary magnesium intake in a national sample of U.S. adults. *J Nutr* 2003;133:2879-82.

Institute of Medicine. Food and Nutrition Board. Dietary Reference Intakes: Calcium, Phosphorus, Magnesium, Vitamin D and Fluoride. National Academy Press. Washington, DC, 1999.

Iseri L, et al. Magnesium: Nature's physiological calcium blocker. *Am Heart J* 108 (1984): 188-93.

Jalali R. Magnesium: The multi-purpose mineral. Article at http://www.mesomorphosis.com/articles/jalali/magnesium.htm

King D, Mainous A 3rd, Geesey M, Woolson R. Dietary magnesium and C-reactive protein levels. *J Am Coll Nutr* 2005 Jun 24(3):166-71.

Kelepouris E and Agus ZS. Hypomagnesemia: Renal magnesium handling. *Semin Nephrol* 1998; 18:58-73.

Li W, Zheng T, Altura BM, Altura BT. Sex steroid hormones exert biphasic effects on cytosolic magnesium ions in cerebral vascular smooth muscle cells: possible relationships to migraine frequency in premenstrual syndromes and stroke incidence. *Brain Res Bull* 2001 Jan 1; 54(1):83-89.

Mauskop A et al. Deficiency in serum ionized magnesium but not total magnesium in patients with migraines. Possible role of ICa2+/IMg2+ ratio. *Headache* 1993 Mar; 33(3): 135-38.

Mauskop A, Altura BM. Role of magnesium in the pathogenesis and treatment of migraines. *Clin Neurosci* 1998; 5:24-27.

Mauskop A et al. Intravenous magnesium sulphate relieves migraine attacks in patients with low serum ionized magnesium levels: a pilot study. *Clin Sci (Lond)* 1994; 89:633-36.

Mauskop A et al. Serum ionized magnesium levels and serum ionized calcium/ionized magneisum ratios in women with menstrual migraine. *Headache* 2002 Apr; 42(4): 242-48.

Naveh-Many T, Epstein E, Silver J. Oestrogens and calcium regulatory hormones: potential implications for bone. *Curr Opin Nephrol Hypertens* 1995 Jul; 4(4): 319-23.

Paolisso G, Scheen A, D'Onofrio F, Lefebvre P. Magnesium and glucose homeostasis. *Diabetologia* 1990; 33:511-14.

Peikert A, Wilimzig C, Kohne-Volland R. Prophylaxis of migraine with oral magnesium:

results from a prospective multi-center, placebo-controlled and double-blind randomized study. *Cephalalgia* June 1996; 16(4): 257-63.

Ramsay LE, Yeo WW, Jackson PR. Metabolic effects of diuretics. *Cardiology* 1994; 84 Suppl 2:48-56.

Rude KR. Magnesium metabolism and deficiency. *Endocrinol Metab Clin North Am* 1993; 22:377-95.

Rude RK. Magnesium deficiency: A cause of heterogeneous disease in humans. *J Bone Miner Res* 1998; 13:749-58.

Saris NE, et al. Magnesium: an update on physiological, clinical, and analytical aspects. *Clinica Chimica Acta* 2000; 294:1-26.

Serfontein WJ. Stress: hormonal and nutrient control. *Natural Medicine* July 2003, issue 9.

Segall L et al. Alterations in the alpha2 isoform of Na,K-ATPase associated with familial hemiplegic migraine type 2. *Proc Nat Acad Sci USA* 2005 Aug 2; 102(31): 11106-11.

Taubert K. Magnesium in migraine: Results of a multicenter pilot study. *Fortschr Med* 1994; 112:328-30.

Tosiello L. Hypomagnesemia and diabetes mellitus. A review of clinical implications. *Arch Intern Med* 1996; 156:1143-48.

US Department of Agriculture, Agricultural Research Service. 2003. USDA National Nutrient Database for Standard Reference, Release 16. Nutrient Data Laboratory Home Page, http://www.nal.usda.gov/fnic/foodcomp.

Walker AF et al. magnesium supplementation alleviates premenstrual symptoms of fluid retention. *J Womens Health* 1998 Nov; 7(9): 1157-65.

Wester P. Magnesium. *Am J Clin Nutr* 45

suppl (1987): 1305-1312.

CHAPTER 9

American Heart Association website; http://www.americanheart.org/presenter.jhtml?identifier=4726

Dzugan SA, Smith AR. Hypercholesterolemia treatment: a new hypothesis or just an accident? *Med Hypotheses* 2002 Dec; 59(6): 751-56.

Kask E. 17-ketosteroids and arteriosclerosis. *Angiology* 1959 Oct; 10:358-68.

Lewis V Hoeger K. Prevention of coronary heart disease: a nonhormonal approach. *Semin Reprod Med* 2005 May; 23(2): 157-66.

Wolfe F, et al. The American College of Rheumatology 1990 criteria for classification of fibromyalgia. *Arthritis Rheum.* 1990 Feb; 33(2):160-72

CHAPTER 10

Adler GK, Manfredsdottir VF, Creskoff KW. Neuroendocrine abnormalities in fibromyalgia. *Curr Pain Headache* Rep 2002 Aug; 6(4):289-98.

Olin R. Fibromyalgia. A neuro-immuno-endocrinologic syndrome? *Lakartidningen* 1995 Feb 22; 92(8):755-8, 761-3.

Rohr UD, Herold J. Melatonin deficiencies in women. *Maturitas* 2002 Apr 15; 41 Suppl 1:S85-104.

Glossary

Adenosine triphosphate (ATP). A compound that transports energy in the cells and is important in the production of RNA. The body produces ATP from food and then ATP produces energy for the body.

Adrenal androgens. The male sex hormones produced by the adrenal gland.

Adrenal cortex. The outer portion of the adrenal gland. It makes up about 80 percent of the gland and is divided into three zones, each one of which is responsible for producing three classes of steroid hormones: glucocorticoids, mineralocorticoids, and adrenal androgens.

Adrenal fatigue. A term used to describe a syndrome that is caused by a decreased ability of the adrenal glands to respond adequately to stress. It is characterized by a wide range of symptoms, including but not limited to chronic fatigue, muscle weakness, overall weakness, frequent headache, cold intolerance, lightheadedness, swollen lymph nodes, and nausea.

Adrenal glands. The two glands located on top of the kidneys. They are mainly responsible for regulating the body's adaptations to physical and emotional stress. Each gland is composed of two

segments: the outer portion (adrenal cortex) and the inner portion (adrenal medulla).

Adrenal medulla. The inner portion of the adrenal gland. It is responsible for producing adrenaline and noradrenaline.

Adreno-corticotropic hormone (ACTH). A hormone manufactured and secreted by the pituitary gland. It stimulates production of cortisol and other adrenal hormones.

Aldosterone. A hormone produced by the adrenal cortex. It is responsible for regulating potassium and sodium levels in the blood and cells, and thus has a significant impact on the amount of fluid in the body's cells.

Androgens. A term that refers to the male sex hormones.

Aura. When referring to migraine, it is a premonition of an attack and is usually characterized by flashing lights, blurry vision, numbness, weakness, difficulty speaking, and hypersensitivity to touch, odors, and/or sound.

Autonomic nervous system. The system that regulates critical functions of the body, including activity of the heart muscle, intestinal tract, and the glands. The autonomic nervous system has two divisions: the sympathetic nervous system and the parasympathetic nervous system.

Bioflavonoids. Nutritional substances that are found in fruits and vegetables that also contain vitamin C.

Bio-identical hormones. Referring to hormones that are derived from plant compounds and are identical to the hormones produced naturally in the human body.

Cholesterol. The most common type of steroid in the body, most of it is manufactured in the liver and other tissues, although some is obtained from diet. Cholesterol is essential to the formation of various hormones (pregnenolone, DHEA, estrogens, progesterone, testosterone, aldosterone, cortisol, corticosterone) as well as vitamin D and bile acids. Cholesterol is present in the blood as lipoproteins: low-density lipoprotein (LDL) and high-density lipoprotein (HDL).

Circadian rhythm. The cyclic fluctuations of hormones and other substances in the body within a twenty-four hour cycle.

Compounding pharmacist. Pharmacist who can create custom medication formulations according to the specifications ordered by a physician. In the case of estrogen, for example, a compounding pharmacist can provide a product composed of varying percentages of estriol, estradiol, and estrone. Compounding pharmacists can also provide you with a drug in a different delivery form; for example, make a liquid of a drug that is normally given as a tablet, which is helpful for individuals who have difficulty swallowing tablets.

Corticotropin-releasing hormone (CRH). A hormone that is secreted by the hypothalamus and which is the main regulator of cortisol production. It also prompts the pituitary to manufacture adreno-corticotropic hormone (ACTH).

Cortisol. The main stress hormone in the body, it is produced by the adrenal cortex.

Dehydroepiandrosterone (DHEA). A hormone produced from pregnenolone and which is a precursor to sex hormones. It is one of the hormones whose levels decline significantly with age and thus is one of the hormones that is restored in the Migraine Cure.

Dihydrotestosterone (DHT). The most potent, naturally occurring male hormone. It is produced from testosterone with the assistance of the enzyme 5-alpha-reductase. Elevated levels of DHT are associated with hair loss (in both men and women), benign prostate hypertrophy, and prostate cancer.

Endocrine glands. Glands that secrete hormones directly into the blood stream and have an impact on metabolism and other body functions. The endocrine gland include the adrenals, hypothalamus, ovaries, pancreas, parathyroid, pineal, pituitary, testicles, thymus, and thyroid.

Estradiol. A type of estrogen, it is produced in the ovaries in women (and in the testes in men) and is the most potent of the naturally occurring estrogens. It is often synthesized and used in hormone replacement therapy. It has many functions, including but not limited to breast development, improving bone density, uterine growth, development of the endometrial lining, adding fat to the hips and breasts during puberty, and accelerating bone maturation.

Estriol. The weakest of the three most common types of estrogen.

Estrogen. Any of several natural substances manufactured by the ovaries, testes, placenta, and certain plants, or produced synthetically, that stimulate the female secondary sex characteristics and prompt menstruation in women. The most common estrogens are estriol, estradiol, and estrone.

Estrone. A type of estrogen, it is weaker than estradiol but more potent than estriol.

Familial hemiplegic migraine. A rare type of hereditary migraine. It is characterized by a migraine attack which is then followed within a day or two by temporary weakness or sensory loss of the limbs on one side of the body, which usually resolves with a few days.

Fibromyalgia. A rheumatic syndrome that is characterized by pain, tenderness, and stiffness of the muscles and tendons and specific tender points on the body. Other symptoms often include chronic fatigue, irritable bowel, sleep disturbances, restless legs, and depression.

5-alpha-reductase. An enzyme that converts testosterone to DHT.

Fructooligosaccharides (FOS). Nondigestible fibers that support and promote friendly bacteria in the gut. They are sometimes referred to as prebiotics because they support probiotics. FOS are found naturally in onions, garlic, and asparagus, and are available in supplement form.

Glucocorticoids. Steroid hormones that are produced in the adrenal cortex. Cortisol is the main natural glucocorticoid.

Homeostasis. The balance of the internal functions and processes of the body.

Hypothalamus. An endocrine gland located in the brain near the pituitary gland. The hypothalamus regulates the majority of the functions of the other endocrine glands, as well as many automatic processes in the body.

Insomnia. A sleep disturbance characterized by an inability to fall asleep, stay asleep, or to get any restorative sleep.

Ion. An atom or a group of atoms that assumes an electrical charge by gaining or losing one or more electrons.

Ion channel. A protein that acts as a pore in a cell membrane and allows certain ions (e.g., calcium ions, magnesium ions, potassium ions) to pass into and out of the cell. When this system malfunctions, many different diseases, collectively known as channelopathies, can occur.

Magnesium. A mineral that is often deficient in humans and one of the main supplements in the Migraine Cure. Magnesium plays important roles in the circadian rhythm and sleep, producing energy from blood sugar, heart health, and many other functions.

Mineralocorticoids. A group of hormones that regulate the balance of electrolytes (ions such as sodium and potassium) and water in the body. Aldosterone is the primary mineralocorticoid.

Nitric oxide. A molecule that is synthesized by oxygen and the amino acid arginine. It dilates the coronary arteries and thus promotes blood flow. It also serves as a neurotransmitter and helps relax the gastrointestinal smooth muscles.

Nociceptor. A receptor for pain that is caused by injury to the body's tissues. Most nociceptors are in the skin or the walls of organs.

Parasympathetic nervous system. A subdivision of the autonomic nervous system, its functions tend to be more calming and relaxing in nature. For example, the parasympathetic nervous system slows heart rate, increases gland activity, and relaxes the sphincter muscles. The parasympathetic nervous system works with the sympathetic nervous system, which tends to have effects that are opposite those of the parasympathetic system.

Phonophobia. A hypersensitivity to sound.

Photophobia. A hypersensitivity to light.

Phytoestrogen. Any one of a group of compounds, found widely in plants, that have weak estrogen properties. Soybeans are a rich source of phytoestrogens.

Pineal gland. An endocrine gland, located deep in the brain, that secretes the hormone melatonin, which regulates the sleep-wake cycle.

Pituitary gland. An endocrine gland, located near the base of the brain, that is often called the master gland because it produces hormones that control many other hormones, including those involved in migraine. The pituitary gland consists of the anterior pituitary, which secretes hormones involved with growth, sexual development, thyroid function, and skin pigmentation; and the posterior pituitary, which secretes hormones involved with uterine contractions and water absorption by the kidneys.

Pluronic lecithin organo (PLO). A gel base used by compounding pharmacists. It is an excellent delivery system for transporting hormones through the skin; it soaks in rapidly and leaves very little residue.

Potassium. The most abundant mineral inside cells. The proper level of potassium is critical for normal cell function, and in imbalance can have serious and deadly affects on the nervous system and heart.

Prebiotics. A type of carbohydrate, called oligosaccharides, that are found naturally in certain fruits and vegetables, including asparagus, bananas, garlic, onions, and tomatoes. Prebiotics are not digested but are transported directly to the gut, where they stimulate the growth of good bacteria, or probiotics. The term was first coined by Professor Glenn Gibson at Reading University and Dr. Marcel Roberfroid of Louvain University, Brussels, in 1995.

Pregnenolone. Sometimes referred to as the "grandmother" of hormones, pregnenolone is a derivative of cholesterol and is a direct precursor for DHEA and progesterone, which in turn are precursors for other hormones, including cortisol, testosterone, and the estrogens.

Probiotics. Supplements that contain healthy or "friendly" bacteria, such as the *Lactobacillus* group, *Bifidobacterium* group, and *Streptococcus thermophilus,* that help maintain healthy intestinal flora and fight the damaging effects of antibiotics.

Prodrome. An early sign or symptom that indicates an impending attack or episode. In migraine this may include flashing lights, blurry vision, feelings of weakness, and/or hypersensitivity to light, odors, and/or sound.

Progesterone. A female hormone, also present in males, that is made primarily by the corpus luteum in the ovary and by the placenta in females, and by the adrenal glands in males. Achieving a balance between progesterone and estrogen is a critical part of the Migraine Cure and overall health as well.

Progestin. Synthetic progesterone.

Prophylactic. Something that serves to prevent or ward off something, especially a disease or symptom.

Saw palmetto. An herb (*Serenoa repens*) that is used to help promote prostate health and to help prevent testosterone from converting into DHT.

Suprachiasmatic nucleus (SCN). Area in the hypothalamus that regulates the circadian rhythms of various processes in the body, including but not limited to sleep-wake, blood pressure, and body temperature.

Sympathetic nervous system. A subdivision of the autonomic nervous system, which performs involuntary functions, the sympathetic nervous system speeds up the heart rate, constricts blood vessels, and raises blood pressure, among other functions. Its activities generally work in synch with and counterbalance those of the parasympathetic nervous system.

Testosterone. A male hormone, also present in small amounts in females, that is produced primarily by the testes in males and possibly by the ovaries and adrenal glands in females. It is responsible for the development of male sexual characteristics, such as a deep voice, body hair, and muscle tone. It is one of the hormones that must be in balance as part of the Migraine Cure.

Vagus nerve. One of the longest nerves in the body, it is a major transmission pathway for chemical and electrical signals between the brain and the gut.

Suggested Reading List

Brownstein, David. *The Miracle of Natural Hormones*. 3rd ed. West Bloomfield, MI: Medical Alternative Press, 2003.

Cherniske, Stephen A. *The DHEA Breakthrough*. Rev. ed. New York: Ballantine, 1998.

Cohen, Jay S., MD. *The Magnesium Solution for Migraine Headaches: The Complete Guide to Using Magnesium to Prevent and Treat Migraine and Cluster Headaches Naturally*. Garden City Park, NY: Square One Publishing, 2004.

Dean, Carolyn, MD. *The Miracle of Magnesium*. New York: Ballantine, 2003.

Dzugan SA, Smith RA. *The simultaneous restoration of neurohormonal and metabolic integrity as a very promising method of migraine management*. Bull Urg Rec Med 2003; 4(4): 622-28.

Hotze SF. Hormones, *Health, and Happiness*. Houston: Forrest Publishing, 2005.

Lee, John R, D. Zava, and Virginia Hopkins. *What Your Doctor May Not Tell You about Breast Cancer*. New York: Warner Books, 2002.

Lee, John R, and Virginia Hopkins. *What Your Doctor May Not Tell You about Menopause*. Rev. and updated. New York: Warner, 2004.

Moore, Neecie, PhD. *The Facts about DHEA*. Arizona: Alethio Corp, 2005.

Oelke, Jane, ND. *Natural Choices for Fibromyalgia*. Stevensville MI: Natural Choices, 2002.

Pierpaoli, Walter. *The Melatonin Miracle*. New York: Pocket Books, 1996.

Regelson, W. *The Super Hormone Promise*. New York: Pocket Books, 1997.

Reiss U. and Martin Zucker. *Natural Hormone Balance for Women: Look Younger, Feel Stronger, and Live Life with Exuberance*. New York: Pocket Books, 2001.

Sahelian, Ray, MD. *Pregnenolone: Nature's Feel Good Hormone*. New York: Avery, 1997.

Seelig, Mildred. *The Magnesium Factor*. New York: Avery, 2003.

Somers, Suzanne. *The Sexy Years: Discover the Hormone Connection: The Secret to Fabulous Sex, Great Health, and Vitality, for Women and Men*. New York: Crown, 2004.

Wilson, James L. *Adrenal Fatigue: The 21st Century Stress Syndrome*. Petaluma, CA: Smart Publications, 2000.

Wright, Jonathan, and John Morganthaler. *Natural Hormone Replacement for Women over 45*. Petaluma, CA: Smart Publications, 1997.

Resources

For More on the Migraine Cure

To participate in or learn more about the Migraine Cure, you can contact the following:

Dr. Sergey Dzugan
1-877-402-2721
www.fountain-migraine.com
The Life Extension Foundation
1-800-226-2370
www.lef.org

Finding a Physician

If you need help finding a physician who prescribes bio-identical hormones and/or blood tests, the following organizations can provide you with names of practitioners in your area. These are not referral services; you are encouraged to check the credentials and backgrounds of any physicians you consider.

American Academy of Anti-Aging Medicine
1510 West Montana Street, Chicago IL 60614
www.worldhealth.net
Click on "find antiaging physicians"

The American College for Advancement in Medicine (ACAM)
23121 Verdugo Drive, Suite 204
Laguna Hills CA 92653
www.acam.org
Click on "Locate an ACAM physician"

American Association for Health Freedom
9912 Georgetown Pike, Suite D-2
Great Falls VA 22066
www.healthfreedom.net
Click on "Find a practitioner"

Compounding Pharmacies

Brister Brothers Pharmacy
1117 Sunset Drive, Suite 102
PO Box 369, Grenada MS 38901
1-800-935-5155
1-662-226-1642
List of compounding pharmacies, by state:
www.project-aware.org/Resource/Pharm.shtml

List (short) of compounding pharmacies at Health World:
http://www.healthy.net/professionals/compound.asp

Provides contact information for local compounding pharmacies:
International Academy of Compounding Pharmacists:
www.iacprx.org
1-800-927-4227

Provides contact information for local compounding pharmacies:
Professional Compounding Centers of America
www.pccarx.com
1-800-331-2498

Sources of hormones and supplements recommended in *The Migraine Cure*:

DHEA and 7-keto-DHEA; Pregnenolone; Progesterone

Life Extension Foundation
1100 W. Commercial Blvd.
Ft. Lauderdale FL 33309
1-800-226-2370
www.lifeextension.com

Organic Pharmacy
PO Box 291, Asheville NC 28802
1-800-819-6742
http://organicpharmacy.org/
manufacturer/Nutricology

Our Health Co-op
931 Village Blvd, Suite 905-480
West Palm Beach Fl 33409
1-561-656-4011
www.ourhealthcoop.com/
A cooperative that supplies supplements
directly to consumers. Tests each production
run of each product and posts results on the
website.

Young Again Nutrients
The Woodlands Center
PO Box 8234, Spring TX 77387-8234
1-877-205-0040
www.youngagain.com

Estrogen, Progesterone, and Testosterone

You will need a prescription from a health-
care professional, which you will need to fill
at a compounding pharmacy. See
"Compounding Pharmacies" for lists of
pharmacies near you.

Magnesium Citrate

Magna-Calm® by Longevity Science
Where To Get It:
Longevity Science/Klabin Marketing
2067 Broadway, Ste. 700
New York NY 10023
1-800-933-9440
www.longevity-
science.net/pages/magnacalm.html

Life Extension (see above)

Probiotic Formula

NutriCology ProGreens
Where To Get It:
Allergy Research Group
2300 North Loop Road
Alameda CA 94502
1-800-545-9960
www.allergyresearchgroup.com

All Nature Pharmaceuticals Inc.
803 Sentous Street
City of Industry CA 91748
1-888-225-7778
www.ihealthtree.com/nutricology.html

Life Extension (see above)

Mother Nature
1-800-439-5506
www.mothernature.com

Organic Pharmacy
(see above)

Our Health Co-op (see above)

Melatonin Formula

Nutribiotic® MetaRest®
Where To Get It:
NutriBiotic
1-800-225-4345
http://store.NutriBiotic.com/
pgi-productspec?2013

Life Extension (see above)

NutriTeam
1-800-785-9791
http://www.nutriteam.com/customer/
product.php?productid=16221

Saw Palmetto and Zinc

Where To Get It:
Life Extension (see above)

Organic Pharmacy (see above)

Parasite Cleansing Program (Unicity™ Paraway® Pack)

Where To Get It:
Life Extension (see above)

Global Mall
http://www.hmglobalmall.com/
unpapafrsh.html
1-866-461-9454

About The Author

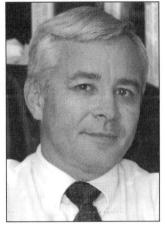

Dr. Sergey A. Dzugan M.D., Ph.D. graduated from the Donetsk State Medical Institute (Ukraine) with a Doctorate of Medicine in 1979. After medical school, he performed his residency in general and cardiovascular surgery and became the Head of Heart Services in 1985. Dr. Dzugan was a distinguished and highly trained educator, physician, and surgeon in the Ukraine.

In 1990, he received his Ph. D. in Medical Science concerning heart rhythm disorder and subsequently became Assistant Professor at the Donetsk State Medical Institute. In May of 1991, he became the first Chief of the Department of Cardiovascular Surgery and Senior Heart Surgeon, in Donetsk District Regional Hospital, Ukraine.

In March of 1993, he became Associate Professor at Donetsk State Medical University. Dr. Dzugan performed a wide spectrum of operations for children and adults, including congenital and acquired heart diseases, and rhythm disorders. As the Head of Heart Surgery he had the highest medical skills and qualifications which can be awarded in his country. As a practicing physician, Dr. Dzugan always found himself more in favor of holistic and natural medicines rather than synthetic. He always believed that strengthening one's immune system would do more to improve health than treating problems after they occur. Because of this, while performing heart surgeries, Dr. Dzugan became more interested in the preventive aspect of heart disease and began studying hormone treatments.

Dr. Dzugan moved to the United States from Ukraine in 1995 and in 1996, became a scientific consultant to Dr. Arnold Smith at the North Central Mississippi Regional Cancer Center in Greenwood, Mississippi. His role there was to stay current on the latest advances in nutriceutical treatments with a particular focus on such to improve immunity and the ability of patients to fight cancer. The North Central Regional Center reviewed his physician extender status by a legal counsel for the Cancer Center, and they were unable to find any objection to this position. In 1998, he has become board certified by the American Board of Anti-Aging Medicine. His employer at the North Central Regional Center has expressed stated that "Dr. Dzugan is extremely valuable to patient care and his role differentiates the North Central Mississippi Regional Cancer Center from that of any other center in the states, because no other center has a full time well qualified staff person to meet the same function." Dr. Smith believes that "Dr. Dzugan is a brilliant, gifted physician whose talents we believe would make a significant contribution to the nation."

In 2001, Dr. Dzugan suggested a new hypothesis of hypercholesterolemia and developed a new statin-free method of high cholesterol treatment. He also developed a unique multimodal program for migraine management.

In 2003 he moved to Ft. Lauderdale, Florida, and became the Manager of the Advisory Department at the Life Extension Foundation. Later, he became President of Life Extension Scientific Information Inc. Dr. Dzugan is a member of the Medical Advisory Board at Life Extension Magazine.

Dr. Dzugan was accepted (June 2006) to the International Academy of Creative Endeavors (Moscow, Russia) as a Corresponding Member of the Academy for his outstanding contribution to the development of new methods of hypercholesterolemia and migraine treatment. He performed presentations multiple times at the prestigious International Congress on Anti-Aging Medicine. The topics of his presentations were "Hypercholesterolemia Treatment: a New Hypothesis or Just an Accident?", "Role of Immunorestorative Therapy in Non Small-Cell Lung Cancer", "A New Method of Migraine Treatment: The Simultaneous

Restoration of Neurohormonal and Metabolic Integrity", and "Hypercholesterolemia Treatment: a New Statin-Free Method". He also was a speaker at the Third Annual Mississippi Partnership for Cancer Control in Underserved Populations Conference. The workshop was titled "Ask the Expert: Questions on Lung Cancer".

Dr. Dzugan is the author of 123 publications in medical journals and these publications include surgical, oncological, academic and anti-aging topics. Also, several articles were published in Life Extension Magazine. He also holds 3 patents in the areas of cardiovascular surgery.

Dr. Dzugan's current primary interests are anti-aging and natural therapy for cholesterol, migraine, fibromyalgia, fatigue, behavioral and hormonal disorders. Since focusing his efforts on Anti-Aging medicine, he has created plans for thousands of patients over the last 8 years, most of which have remained on their plans.

Index

vous systems, 38, 39–42
  autonomic nervous system and, 38, 39
  balance between, 19, 38, 39–42, 59, 92, 107
  digestive system and, 107
  functioning of, 39
  opposing actions of, 41
symptomatic drug treatment, 49, 52, 53
synthetic hormones, 62–63, 80, 164–166, 173–174

T

testosterone, 83–88
  case study about, 85–88
  optimal vs. reference ranges of, 35
  production of, 83–84
  as steroid hormone, 28, 31, 32, 34
  taking of, 84–85, 166–167
  testing for, 84
therapy. *See* treatment
treatment. *See also* Migraine cure
  alternative approaches to, 5, 53
  case studies of, 133–144
  cost of, 5, 164, 166
  current approaches to, 43–44, 45–48, 49–53
  drugs used in, 2–3, 5, 11, 12–14, 44, 49–53, 134, 138
  effectiveness of, 43–44, 45–48, 49–53, 134, 138
  hormone restoration therapy. *See* hormone restoration therapy

melatonin and, 96–97
triggers (for migraines), 6–8
  definition of, 4–5
  food as, 6, 54, 118
  sleep as, 93
  types of, 6–8
triptans, 2, 11. *See also* drug treatment

V

vagus nerve, 113–114
vitamin B6, 103–104
vomiting, 2, 3, 23

W

weather (as migraine trigger), 7
WHI. *See* Women's Health Initiative
women
  heart disease among, 150
  hormone production of, 7, 31, 84
  hormone replacement therapy for. *See* hormone replacement therapy
  menopause and, 45, 48, 58, 79, 81, 101
  menstruation and, 7, 10, 45, 59, 74, 79, 126
  pregnancy and, 7, 45
  prevalence of migraines among, 5, 8, 10, 45, 59
Women's Health Initiative (WHI), 46, 71

Z

zinc, 89

How to stay informed of the latest advances in diet and nutrition:

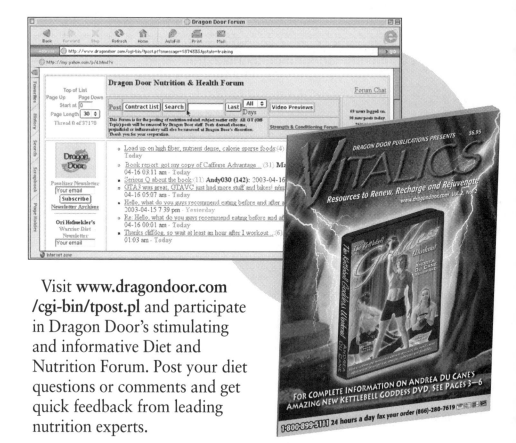

Visit **www.dragondoor.com /cgi-bin/tpost.pl** and participate in Dragon Door's stimulating and informative Diet and Nutrition Forum. Post your diet questions or comments and get quick feedback from leading nutrition experts.

Visit **www.dragondoor.com** and browse the Articles section and other pages for groundbreaking theories and products for improving your health and well being.

Call Dragon Door Publications at **1-800-899-5111** and request your FREE Vitalics catalog of fitness books, videos, supplements and equipment.

ORDERING INFORMATION

Complete and mail with full payment to: Dragon Door Publications, P.O. Box 1097, West Chester, OH 45071

Please print clearly

Sold To: A

Name_____

Street_____

City_____

State_____ Zip_____

Day phone*_____

* Important for clarifying questions on orders

Please print clearly

SHIP TO: *(Street address for delivery)*   B

Name_____

Street_____

City_____

State_____ Zip_____

Email_____

Warning to foreign customers:
The Customs in your country may or may not tax or otherwise charge you an additional fee for goods you receive. Dragon Door Publications is charging you only for U.S. handling and international shipping. Dragon Door Publications is in no way responsible for any additional fees levied by Customs, the carrier or any other entity.

Warning!
This may be the last issue of the catalog you receive.

If we rented your name, or you haven't ordered in the last two years you may not hear from us again. If you wish to stay informed about products and services that can make a difference to your health and well-being, please indicate below.

Name_____

Address_____

City_____ State_____

Zip_____

Item #	Qty.	Item Description	Item Price	A or B	Total

HANDLING AND SHIPPING CHARGES · NO COD'S
Total Amount of Order Add:

$00.00 to $24.99 add $5.00	$100.00 to $129.99 add $12.00
$25.00 to $39.99 add $6.00	$130.00 to $169.99 add $14.00
$40.00 to $59.99 add $7.00	$170.00 to $199.99 add $16.00
$60.00 to $99.99 add $10.00	$200.00 to $299.99 add $18.00
	$300.00 and up add $20.00

Canada & Mexico add $8.00. All other countries triple U.S. charges.

Total of Goods	
Shipping Charges	
Rush Charges	
Kettlebell Shipping Charges	
OH residents add 6% sales tax	
MN residents add 6.5% sales tax	
TOTAL ENCLOSED	

Do You Have A Friend Who'd Like To Receive This Catalog?

We would be happy to send your friend a free copy. Make sure to print and complete in full:

Name_____

Address_____

City_____ State_____

Zip_____

METHOD OF PAYMENT ___CHECK ___M.O. ___MASTERCARD ___VISA ___DISCOVER ___AMEX

Account No. *(Please indicate all the numbers on your credit card)*   EXPIRATION DATE

☐☐☐☐ ☐☐☐☐ ☐☐☐☐ ☐☐☐☐   ☐☐/☐☐

Day Phone ( )_____

SIGNATURE_____ DATE_____

NOTE: We ship best method available for your delivery address. Foreign orders are sent by air. Credit card or International M.O. only. For rush processing of your order, add an additional $10.00 per address. Available on money order & charge card orders only.

Errors and omissions excepted. Prices subject to change without notice.

ORDERING INFORMATION

Customer Service Questions? Please call us between 9:00am– 11:00pm EST Monday to Friday at 1-800-899-5111. Local and foreign customers call 513-346-4160 for orders and customer service

100% One-Year Risk-Free Guarantee. If you are not completely satisfied with any product–for any reason, no matter how long after you received it–we'll be happy to give you a prompt exchange, credit, or refund, as you wish. Simply return your purchase to us, and please let us know why you were dissatisfied–it will help us to provide better products and services in the future. *Shipping and handling fees are non-refundable.*

Telephone Orders For faster service you may place your orders by calling Toll Free 24 hours a day, 7 days a week, 365 days per year. When you call, please have your credit card ready.

1·800·899·5111
24 HOURS A DAY
FAX YOUR ORDER (866) 280-7619

Complete and mail with full payment to: Dragon Door Publications, P.O. Box 1097, West Chester, OH 45071

Please print clearly

Sold To: A

Name_____

Street_____

City_____

State_____ Zip_____

Day phone*_____

* *Important for clarifying questions on orders*

Please print clearly

SHIP TO: *(Street address for delivery)*   B

Name_____

Street_____

City_____

State_____ Zip_____

Email_____

Item #	Qty.	Item Description	Item Price	A or B	Total

HANDLING AND SHIPPING CHARGES • NO COD'S

Total Amount of Order Add:

$00.00 to $24.99 add $5.00	$100.00 to $129.99 add $12.00
$25.00 to $39.99 add $6.00	$130.00 to $169.99 add $14.00
$40.00 to $59.99 add $7.00	$170.00 to $199.99 add $16.00
$60.00 to $99.99 add $10.00	$200.00 to $299.99 add $18.00
	$300.00 and up add $20.00

Canada & Mexico add $8.00. All other countries triple U.S. charges.

Total of Goods	
Shipping Charges	
Rush Charges	
Kettlebell Shipping Charges	
OH residents add 6% sales tax	
MN residents add 6.5% sales tax	
Total Enclosed	

Method of Payment ___Check ___M.O. ___Mastercard ___Visa ___Discover ___Amex

Account No. *(Please indicate all the numbers on your credit card)*   EXPIRATION DATE

☐☐☐☐ ☐☐☐☐ ☐☐☐☐ ☐☐☐☐   ☐☐/☐☐

Day Phone ( )_____

SIGNATURE_____ DATE _____

NOTE: We ship best method available for your delivery address. Foreign orders are sent by air. Credit card or International M.O. only. For rush processing of your order, add an additional $10.00 per address. Available on money order & charge card orders only.

Errors and omissions excepted. Prices subject to change without notice.

Warning to foreign customers:
The Customs in your country may or may not tax or otherwise charge you an additional fee for goods you receive. Dragon Door Publications is charging you only for U.S. handling and international shipping. Dragon Door Publications is in no way responsible for any additional fees levied by Customs, the carrier or any other entity.

Warning!
This may be the last issue of the catalog you receive.

If we rented your name, or you haven't ordered in the last two years you may not hear from us again. If you wish to stay informed about products and services that can make a difference to your health and well-being, please indicate below.

Name_____

Address_____

City_____ State_____

Zip_____

Do You Have A Friend Who'd Like To Receive This Catalog?

We would be happy to send your friend a free copy. Make sure to print and complete in full:

Name_____

Address_____

City_____ State_____

Zip_____   DDP 11/06